The Manhattan Diaries Series

Central Park's Fitness Hacks

How NYC's Best Shape Up

Manhattan Vitality
Just Like That

The Manhattan Diaries Series

Manhattan Allure – Just Like That

Manhattan Vitality – Just Like That

Manhattan Lifestyle – Just Like That

Manhattan Ambition – Just Like That

The Manhattan Diaries Series

Central Park's Fitness Hacks

How NYC's Best Shape Up

Manhattan Vitality
Just Like That

CANDICE MALONE

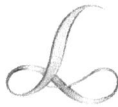

Urban Chronicles Publishing House
an imprint of The Ridge Publishing Group
Coeur d'Alene, Idaho, U.S.A.

DISCLAIMER: The ideas, concepts, and opinions expressed in The Manhattan Diaries Series (hereinafter referred to as "Series") are intended to help readers make thoughtful and informed decisions about their lifestyle. This Series is sold with the understanding that author and publisher are not rendering medical advice of any kind, nor is this Series intended to replace the medical advice, nor to diagnose, prescribe, or treat any disease, condition, illness, or injury. It should not be used as a substitute for treatment by or the advice of a professional healthcare provider. It is recommended that before beginning any diet or exercise program, including any aspect of the Series, you receive full medical clearance from a licensed healthcare provider. Although the author and publisher have endeavored to ensure that the information provided in the Series is complete and accurate, the author and publisher claim no responsibility to any person or entity for any liability, loss, or damage caused or alleged to be caused directly or indirectly as a result of the use, application, or interpretation of the material in this Series, or any errors or omissions in the Series.

CREDIT: This book was written with limited assistance of ChatGPT, an AI language model developed by OpenAI. The collaboration provided unique insights and support in crafting content. The book cover was created using Midjourney tools and Adobe Photoshop, ensuring a visually captivating design.

Library of Congress Control Number: 2024923938

Central Park's Fitness Hacks: How NYC's Best Shape Up by Candice Malone

ISBN: 978-1-956905-49-6 (e-book)
ISBN: 978-1-956905-48-9 (Softcover)

1. Health & Fitness / Exercise. 2. Health & Fitness / Healthy Living. 3. Self-Help / Motivational & Inspirational. 4. Self-Help / Personal Growth / Happiness. 5. Sports & Recreation / Running & Jogging. 6. Health & Fitness / Weight Loss. I. Title. II. Series.

First Edition: October 2024
Printed in the United States of America

Contents

The Manhattan Diaries Series

DARE TO REIMAGINE YOURSELF . . .

21 Steps to Reinvent and Discover a Side of You Manhattan's Never Seen

The Manhattan Diaries Series presents:

Manhattan Allure—Just Like That mini-series (books 1–5)

Manhattan Vitality—Just Like That mini-series (books 6–10)

Manhattan Lifestyle—Just Like That mini-series (books 11–16)

Manhattan Ambition—Just Like That mini-series (books 17–21)

Meet the Author

https://www.LAMoeszinger.com

Meet the Publisher, Urban Chronicles Publishing House

https://www.NewYouniversityChronicles.com

Step into the whirlwind world of New York's glitzy underbelly, where the scintillating secrets and laugh-out-loud confessions of a metropolitan woman are laid bare by someone truly in the know. Through essays pulled from her chic "Manhattanite's Survival Guide—Success in the City," L invites us on an unforgettable strut from her glamorous youth, through her middle-aged mazes, and into her fabulous sixties.

For the juiciest tidbits about L's life, her "Manhattan Chronicles" blog is the place to be. This blog is an unfiltered dive into L's world, from her spiritual musings to her meticulous weigh-ins to her New Youniversity Chronicles—The Manhattan Diaries series—personal tales. Dive into her cosmos at her blog site: https://www.ManhattanChronicles.com.

The Manhattan Diaries Series

Central Park's Fitness Hacks

How NYC's Best Shape Up

Manhattan Vitality
Just Like That

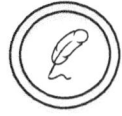

Introduction: From Skyline Views to Sculpted Moves – Central Park's Best-Kept Fitness Secrets

Hey there, fitness fanatics and urban explorers! As you roam the vibrant streets of New York City, have you ever wondered how the city's fittest maintain their enviable physiques amid the bustling metropolis? Do you jog through Central Park with the confidence of a true New Yorker, or are you still piecing together the secrets of getting in shape like NYC's finest? Well, darlings, the city holds the key to fitness excellence, and I'm here to spill the beans in "Central Park's Fitness Hacks: How NYC's Best Shape Up."

In this invigorating journey, I'm taking you behind the scenes of Manhattan's fitness aficionados. Success in the Big Apple isn't just about wit or navigating its concrete canyons—it's about sculpting a body that turns heads and leaves a lasting impression at every chic event, from uptown runs to downtown workouts. I've mingled with the city's fitness elites, sweated through countless classes, and uncovered the fitness secrets that keep Manhattan's finest looking and feeling their absolute best. But remember, true fitness begins from within.

Consider this your VIP invitation to a limited-edition of The Manhattan Diaries series, fitness experience. Whether you savor this fitness treasure trove over leisurely workouts, dive into it week by week, or read it while stretching in Central Park, the pace is entirely up to you. Picture yourself diving into a chapter with your morning workout or immersing yourself in the entire book during a fitness weekend getaway. Within these pages, you'll unlock the keys to becoming the master of your fitness destiny, and the vitality that follows will leave you revitalized.

As we embark on this journey together, I'll be your fitness confidante, revealing how effortlessly you can shape up like a pro in the city that never sleeps. This guide isn't just about fitness tips; it's a rejuvenation of your spirit, your relationships, and your fitness aspirations in the city. Join me in uncovering the secrets that will allow you to sculpt a body that radiates confidence and health, just like a Manhattanite on a Central Park jog. I'm not just dedicated to helping you master the art of fitness; I'm here to ignite the wellness in your heart that propels you to your most vibrant self. Embrace it, and the energy of New York will be yours to command!

My passion for this city-centric guide is born from my own personal fitness journey, filled with highs and lows, fitness addiction, and moments of revelation. Like many city dwellers, I had to navigate the fitness maze, sometimes veering off the well-trodden path. But today, I stand before you, ready to inspire you to shape up like a pro in the city, with your workout gear in hand.

As time sails on the Hudson River, our life paths inevitably intersect. For me, the whirlwind of career pursuits, downtown fitness classes, and self-discovery converged with my love for the city, leading me to work with the Urban Chronicles Publishing House.

New York City's fitness allure isn't limited to celebrities or trust fund beneficiaries; it's accessible to everyone, whether you're a fitness enthusiast in your twenties or a seasoned athlete in your sixties. Embrace this journey with me as we embark on a path to city stardom in this seventh step—The Manhattan Diaries series is a twenty-one step journey; twenty-one books to reinvent and discover a side of you Manhattan's never met.

"Central Park's Fitness Hacks" equips you with the tools to not only work up a sweat but also to sculpt a physique that's red-carpet ready. I'm here as your city guardian, ensuring you realize that everything you crave starts within. Elevate your fitness game with Manhattan's finest fitness secrets, and watch as your wellness, vitality, and maybe even your dream partner, follow suit. If you've got fitness dreams of shaping up like a pro, this guide is your key to unlocking them! I've witnessed friends rise to fitness stardom, proving that as you align within, the city will reflect it back in strength, confidence, and health. That's a promise straight from the heart of New York.

Relying on The Manhattan Diaries series has always been my compass. Whenever the city threw a fitness curveball my way, this guide, in The Manhattan Diaries series, steered me right back to my path of vitality. The allure of always being in peak shape keeps me coming back to these pages, and trust me, it's far more exhilarating that settling for mediocrity.

With every page you turn, you'll discover the blueprint, insider fitness secrets, and the support you need to make your fitness journey an exhilarating adventure. This series is tailored for everyone, from those seeking a fabulous fitness career to social butterflies and wellness empire builders.

There are countless ways to rise in the Big Apple, but if you're looking for the chicest route to excellence, it's right here in The Manhattan Diaries. Immerse yourself in its treasures while reciting positive mantras, and let the city's vibrancy chase away any doubts; and, in this case, allowing you to shape up like a pro and live your most active life.

Navigating the City with The Manhattan Diaries

Welcome to "Central Park's Fitness Hacks: How NYC's Best Shape Up." Think of this edition of The Manhattan Diaries as your personal cosmopolitan fitness diary, as interactive as an invitation to Manhattan's most exclusive wellness gatherings. Each chapter is enriched with journal pages, waiting for your Manhattan musings and anecdotes. Whether you want to record the day's highlights in your "Fitness Chronicles" or delve into deep reflections in your "Fitness Confessions," these pages are yours to fill—see Cocktails and Chronicles: "Journal Pages: Pen Your Tales."

But . . .

CENTRAL PARK'S FITNESS HACKS

1 Before you start penning your thoughts, take a moment to breathe. Close your eyes and, in that quiet moment, express a heartfelt "thank you" to the city that never sleeps. Feel that rush of gratitude, as if you've just completed a Central Park run with the city's skyline as your backdrop. Let that "thank you" resonate deep within your heart—because that, my dear readers, is the magic of Manhattan.

2 Begin by detailing the fabulous strides you've made since delving into the last glamorous fitness advice you've received. Write them down under "Completed Tasks," and revel in the feeling of conquering every workout, like a true fitness pro.

3 Once you've celebrated your fitness triumphs, turn the page to "Action Items" and outline your wellness aspirations. Reflect on what's left to conquer in your fitness journey, capturing your next steps in this transformational saga.

Through The Manhattan Diaries series, you'll encounter timeless "inspirational quotes" that are as iconic as Manhattan's skyline. These pearls of wisdom are your city mantras. Savor them, recite each word as if you're celebrating a personal best in Central Park, and let them resonate deep within your urban fitness soul.

As you approach the end of each guide, you'll discover a "City Roundup." Here, you'll find a chic recap summarizing all the insider tips, in this case, from your fitness escapade, ensuring you never miss a New York fitness minute.

So, get ready to shape up like an A-lister, darlings. Behind the cityscape lies a world of fitness glamour, strength, and endless possibilities for your physique. It's time to work up a sweat, sculpt your body, and live your most vibrant life in the city that never sleeps.

Central Park's Fitness Hacks: How NYC's Best Shape Up

Darlings, slip into those designer sneakers and embrace the allure of Central Park. The seventh enticing entry in The Manhattan Diaries series has arrived: "Central Park's Fitness Hacks: How NYC's Best Shape Up."

Imagine the stories those winding paths and serene meadows could tell, if only they could talk! From runway models to Upper East Side mavens, Central Park isn't just New York's lungs—it's its pulsating heart and sculpted muscles, too.

Oh, sweethearts, a life in Manhattan is nothing short of cinematic, and this isn't just about attending the right parties or snagging the latest couture. It's about dancing to the rhythm of your heartbeat, chasing after the city's brisk pace, and strengthening your core amidst skyscrapers and starry dreams. Dive into fitness hacks that are more than just routines—they're life-savers! Sidestep heart troubles, waltz past diabetes, and pirouette around certain cancers. Not to mention, the afterglow: fewer stress lines and more genuine smiles.

"Central Park's Fitness Hacks: How NYC's Best Shape Up," with its sylvan secrets, is your ticket to not just looking, but feeling like Manhattan royalty. Come, break a sweat with the city's elite and discover the true path to a remarkable life. Strap up, laces tied, and let's get that heart racing!

Meet the Maestros Behind the Curtain

Welcome to the glittering realm of The Manhattan Diaries series, penned by an eclectic group of scribes who know how to make words shimmer just like that Midtown skyline. Each of these writers possesses the kind of Manhattan moxie that's as electrifying as a Saturday night at Studio 54. Picture the literary equivalent of the fabulous foursome from "Sex and the City," but with a little extra Manhattan mascara.

Our authors, darlings, aren't just writers; they're connoisseurs of all things NYC, dishing out stories with the precision of a Fifth Avenue stylist crafting the perfect blowout. Their tales are imbued with the kind of insider knowledge only those who've sipped martinis at the city's most secretive spots can truly understand.

So, as you delve into the pages of The Manhattan Diaries know that you're not just reading words, you're sipping on the prose of New York's finest literary mixologists. Here's to a journey as sparkling and unforgettable as a New York night out. Cheers, darling!

Behind the Scenes with the Urban Chronicles Publishing House

In the whirlwind of New York's high society, the Urban Chronicles Publishing House has emerged as the ultimate style sage for modern-day self-help. Over a cosmopolitan-fueled decade, they've become the city's go-to curators for crafting that sought-after, enviable life. The Manhattan Diaries? Envision it as your exclusive, VIP backstage pass, dripping with Upper East Side allure.

If you've ever pictured yourself sashaying through Manhattan with poise, if you've craved that skyline backdrop to your impeccable life, or if you simply seek the secrets whispered in the plush corners of the city's most exclusive clubs—The Manhattan Diaries is your ticket. Crafted under the elite banner, Urban Chronicles Publishing House, this imprint doesn't just offer you insights; it's your personal invite to the city's most glamorous circles.

> ➢ **Forever en Vogue**. Everyone, from the Wall Street moguls to the aspiring Broadway stars, dreams of basking in New York's radiant glow, of living a life drenched in style and substance. The wisdom in The Manhattan Diaries is as timeless as a Fifth Avenue romance, ensuring you're always en vogue.

➢ **A Blueprint for the Elite**. Nestled within these pages are the golden rules of city living, from mastering the cocktail chatter to undergoing a dazzling reinvention. Whether you're a seasoned socialite, an ambitious parent, or a fresh-eyed dreamer, these guides have something to make your heart race a little faster.

➢ **The Perfect Accessory**. Their petite stature makes these guides a seamless fit for your Prada clutch or your gym tote. Think of them as your urban survival kit—a blend of wisdom and wit that's as crucial as your red lipstick for those Manhattan nights.

Take a sip of this rich concoction, and let the Urban Chronicles Publishing House unlock Manhattan, unveiling a New York you only dreamed of. Welcome to the allure of the elite, darling.

Unveiling The Ridge Publishing Group

Picture The Ridge Publishing Group as the rising star on New York's literary and entertainment horizon. Envision an eclectic empire—books, cinema, and board games—setting the stage to become the world's haute couture of theological discourse. Think Fifth Avenue for theological resources: luxurious, elite, and unparalleled.

Dive into their esteemed collections. They hold the keys to the illustrious Guardians of Biblical Truth Publishing Group and the evocative New Narrated Study Bible (NNSB) series. Delve deeper and find the Hoyle Theology Publishing Group and its opulent Hoyle Theology Encyclopedia—a treasure trove for the cerebral sophisticate. And for those who like their theology paired with a cinematic flair, there's the Documentaries in Print Publishing Group with its tantalizing series like Defending the Faith. And, of course, for those cocktail nights with a side of divine strategy, the Heaven's Seminary board games and card decks offer a chic twist.

But that's not all. The Ridge Publishing Group is more than a theological publishing powerhouse; it's a brand. Alongside its flagship, it flaunts trendy imprints: AuthorsDoor Group and AuthorsDoor Leadership (check them out at the glamorous digital boulevard of https://www.AuthorsDoor.com), the ritzy Urban Chronicles Publishing House and New Youniversity (make your reservation at https://www.LAMoeszinger.com), and the novel delights of Ethan Fox Books (sip your martini and browse https://www.EthanFox Books.com).

For a sneak peek into the world where theology meets Manhattan glamour, rendezvous at their digital penthouse: https://www.Ridge PublishingGroup.com. It's theology made chic.

A NOTE TO THE READER

Typos in this book? Errors (and inconsistencies) can get through proofreaders, so if you do find any typos or grammatical errors in this book, I'd be very grateful if you could let me know using this email address typos@LAMoeszinger.com. Thank you ☺

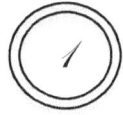

1

The Bethesda Bootcamp: Sculpting Dreams by the Terrace

Manhattan, a city that doesn't just shimmer in its glamorous attire—it pulses, vibrant and alive, as each resident contributes to its breathtaking narrative. Stories of dreams, diligence, and the sheer will to become the best version of oneself. And in this sprawling urban jungle, where the game is ever-changing, it isn't about how many miles you run, but how you run those miles—with tenacity, grace, and an unyielding spirit.

Now imagine: You're pacing alongside Bethesda Terrace, with Central Park's natural opulence as your backdrop. The world doesn't notice the brand of your sneakers; instead, they're enchanted by the dedication in your eyes. That, darling, is the Bethesda Burn, an art form that speaks of commitment, of molding oneself just as a sculptor would with clay—delicately, diligently, and with a dash of drama.

In this invigorating chapter of The Manhattan Diaries, we dive deep into the rituals of the Bethesda Bootcamp. From the heart-racing highs of the hill sprints to the meditative calm of cool-down stretches under the arches, you'll learn the secrets to honing not just the body, but the soul.

But let's be clear: This isn't merely about sculpted abs or toned limbs. Oh no. It's about sculpting dreams, carving out moments of reflection amidst the relentless hustle. It's about charging forward with an intent, with a mission, amidst the verdant vistas of Central Park, embracing both its tranquility and its challenges.

So, walk with me—better yet, sprint! Let's feel the rhythm of the city beneath our feet, each drop of sweat a testament to our resolve. Because, sweetheart, in Manhattan, every workout is an ode to self-love and ambition. Lace up those trainers and let's embark on a transformative journey, for the city doesn't just witness your effort—it applauds it. Welcome to The

Manhattan Diaries—where your determination can be as iconic as the city's skyline.

The Art of the Bethesda Burn: Unleash Your Inner Sculptor

Darlings, in the heart of Manhattan, there's a fitness experience that's more than just exercise; it's an art form. Welcome to "The Art of the Bethesda Burn: Unleash Your Inner Sculptor." Picture yourself on the Bethesda Terrace, surrounded by the vibrant energy of Central Park. Here, we'll explore the secrets of sculpting not only your body but your dreams. It's a journey of commitment, ambition, and finding serenity amidst the city's hustle and bustle. Now, let's dive in, shall we?

➢ **Sculpting Your Body, Sculpting Your Dreams**: This isn't your average workout; it's a transformative journey. The Bethesda Burn is about molding your body just like a sculptor with clay-delicately, diligently, and with a dash of drama.

➢ **The Pulse of Central Park**: Central Park is more than just a park; it's your fitness playground. Imagine sprinting alongside the Bethesda Terrace with the park's natural opulence as your backdrop. It's not about how many miles you run, but how you run them-with tenacity, grace, and an unyielding spirit.

➢ **Hill Sprints and Archway Zen**: Experience the heart-pounding highs of hill sprints and the meditative calm of cool-down stretches under the iconic arches. It's a unique blend of exhilaration and introspection that defines the Bethesda Bootcamp.

➢ **Tranquil Moments in a Bustling City**: Amidst the relentless hustle of Manhattan, the Bethesda Bootcamp offers you precious moments of reflection. It's about finding inner calm while surrounded by the vivacious energy of the city.

- ➢ **The Rhythm of the City Beneath Your Feet**: Feel the pulse of Manhattan beneath your trainers as you sprint along the city streets. It's not just a workout; it's a rhythmic dance with the urban jungle that encourages you to push your limits.

- ➢ **Lace-Up, Show-Up, Level-Up**: With each workout, you're not just shaping your physique; you're leveling up in the game of life. The Bethesda Burn instills a sense of commitment that transcends fitness and seeps into every aspect of your journey.

- ➢ **The City Applauds Your Effort**: In Manhattan, your determination is celebrated as much as any Broadway show or world-famous landmark. The city doesn't just witness your effort; it applauds it with every stride you take.

- ➢ **An Iconic Journey**: Your journey through the Bethesda Bootcamp is as iconic as the skyline of Manhattan itself. Just as the city rises high, so does your determination, ambition, and the desire to become the best version of yourself.

- ➢ **Strength in Unity: Sweating Together, Rising Together**: The Bethesda Burn isn't a solo journey; it's a shared experience. Surrounded by fellow New Yorkers, each stride and stretch builds a sense of unity, fueling your energy and reminding you that in Manhattan, resilience is a collective spirit.

As we conclude this chapter, my dears, remember that the Bethesda Burn is more than just a fitness routine—it's an ode to self-love and ambition. In Manhattan, where every corner tells a story, this experience becomes an integral part of the city's narrative. So, join me in sculpting dreams and embracing the city's heartbeat as you unleash your inner sculptor. In the heart of Manhattan, every journey, whether it's through fitness or life itself, is as iconic as the city's skyline, a skyline that's intertwined with the dreams and aspirations of its spirited residents.

Completed Tasks: Inner Sculptor Activities

Inspirational Quote

IF YOU CAN DREAM IT, YOU CAN DO IT. — Walt Disney

Action Items: Intentions and Thoughts

From Hill Sprints to Archway Zen: The Rituals of Bethesda Bootcamp

Darlings, join me as we embark on a journey through the heart-pounding rituals of the Bethesda Bootcamp in the heart of Manhattan. From exhilarating hill sprints to moments of serene reflection under the iconic arches, this chapter is a deep dive into the unique fitness experience that this city offers. It's about more than just exercise; it's about sculpting not only your body but your soul amidst the vibrant energy of Central Park. So, let's explore "From Hill Sprints to Archway Zen: The Rituals of Bethesda Bootcamp" together.

➤ **Heart-Pounding Hill Sprints**: Imagine racing up the rolling hills of Central Park, feeling your heart pound with each step. It's not just a workout; it's a thrilling challenge that pushes you to new heights and tests your limits.

➤ **The Bethesda Terrace Backdrop**: The Bethesda Terrace provides a breathtaking backdrop for your fitness journey. With its iconic arches and serene atmosphere, it's the perfect place to find your inner zen after an intense workout.

➤ **Cool-Down Stretches Under the Arches**: After the adrenaline rush of hill sprints, find moments of tranquility under the arches. Cool-down stretches become a meditative experience, allowing you to reflect and rejuvenate amidst the hustle of the city.

➤ **Embracing the Park's Natural Opulence**: Central Park's lush greenery and shimmering waters create a natural oasis in the heart of Manhattan. It's a setting that inspires and rejuvenates, making every workout feel like an escape into a world of natural opulence.

➤ **Community and Camaraderie**: The Bethesda Bootcamp isn't just about fitness; it's about forging connections with fellow fitness enthusiasts. It's a place where you can share stories, support one another, and find a sense of community in the bustling city.

➤ **Cultivating Mind-Body Balance**: Hill sprints challenge your physical limits, while cool-down stretches under the arches cultivate mind-body balance. It's a holistic approach to wellness that leaves you feeling invigorated and centered.

➤ **Unearthing Inner Strength**: The Bethesda Bootcamp is not just about sculpting your body; it's about unearthing your inner strength and resilience. It's a reminder that you are capable of achieving greatness, both in fitness and in life.

➤ **Unearthing Inner Strength**: The Bethesda Bootcamp is not just about sculpting your body; it's about unearthing your inner strength and resilience. It's a reminder that you are capable of achieving greatness, both in fitness and in life.

➤ **A Journey of Self-Discovery**: Each ritual of the Bethesda Bootcamp is a step on a transformative journey of self-discovery. Just as Manhattan's landmarks tell stories of ambition and dreams, your journey through these rituals is a testament to your own unique narrative.

As we conclude this chapter, my dears, remember that the rituals of the Bethesda Bootcamp are not just about physical fitness; they're about mental and emotional wellness. Just as Manhattan's skyline is a masterpiece of ambition and determination, your journey through the Bethesda Bootcamp is a testament to your own dedication and inner strength. It's a journey that blends the highs of challenge with the soothing calm of reflection, much like the juxtaposition of bustling city streets and the tranquil arches of the Bethesda Terrace.

Completed Tasks: Bootcamp Ritual Activities

Inspirational Quote

LIFE IS 10 PERCENT WHAT HAPPENS TO YOU AND 90 PERCENT HOW YOU REACT TO IT. — Charles R. Swindoll

Action Items: Intentions and Thoughts

Central Park: Your Fitness Playground

Darlings, picture yourself in the heart of Manhattan, where the bustling cityscape gives way to the tranquil oasis of Central Park. It's not just a park; it's your ultimate fitness playground. Welcome to "Central Park: Your Fitness Playground." In this chapter, we'll explore how this iconic green haven becomes the backdrop for your fitness journey, offering you more than just exercise —it's a chance to sculpt dreams and find moments of serenity amidst the city's vibrant energy.

> ➢ **An Urban Escape**: Central Park is your sanctuary in the midst of Manhattan's hustle and bustle. Step into this urban oasis and leave the city's chaos behind as you embark on your fitness adventure.

> ➢ **The Bethesda Terrace Magic**: The Bethesda Terrace, with its majestic arches and shimmering waters, serves as the epicenter of your fitness experience. It's a place where dreams are carved just as elegantly as the park's iconic sculptures.

> ➢ **Running the Central Park Loop**: The Central Park Loop, with its winding pathways and stunning views, is your fitness track. Every step you take here is an ode to self-love and ambition, as you embrace the challenges of the course.

> ➢ **Sculpting Dreams Amongst Nature**: Central Park's lush greenery, tranquil lakes, and diverse flora provide the perfect backdrop for not just your fitness journey, but also for moments of reflection and self-discovery.

> ➢ **Cultural and Artistic Inspirations**: Beyond fitness, Central Park offers a wealth of cultural and artistic experiences. From open-air concerts to art installations, it's a place where creativity flourishes, inspiring your own journey towards self-expression.

➢ **Meeting Point for Kindred Spirits**: Central Park isn't just for solo fitness enthusiasts; it's a place where kindred spirits gather. You'll find communities of runners, yogis, and fitness enthusiasts who share your passion for health and well-being.

➢ **Serenity Amidst the City's Pulse**: Amidst the city's constant hustle, Central Park offers moments of serenity. Whether it's practicing yoga by the reservoir or meditating beneath the Bow Bridge, it's a space where you can find inner peace.

➢ **A Haven for Dreams and Aspirations**: Central Park, like Manhattan's iconic landmarks, is a place where dreams are nurtured and aspirations take flight. Your fitness journey here is a reflection of your desire to rise above the ordinary and achieve greatness.

➢ **Sunrise Workouts with Skyline Views**: Start your day with sunrise workouts along Central Park's eastern edges, where the morning light illuminates the skyline and fuels your motivation. With each breath, you're reminded of the city's energy, embracing both the quiet dawn and the rising pulse of Manhattan.

➢ **Seasons of Strength**: Central Park transforms with each season, adding a new layer to your fitness journey. From winter's invigorating chill to spring's fresh blooms, each workout becomes a celebration of resilience and renewal, keeping your goals in step with nature's rhythm.

In the heart of Manhattan, where dreams are as enduring as the city's towering skyscrapers and landmarks represent the spirit of ambition, Central Park stands as a testament to nature's harmony with human endeavor. Embrace it, my darlings, and let it be your fitness playground and sanctuary, where every moment becomes a chance to sculpt your dreams and discover the essence of your extraordinary journey.

Completed Tasks: Park Fitness Playground Activities

Inspirational Quote

SET YOUR GOALS HIGH, AND DON'T STOP TILL YOU GET THERE. — Bo
Jackson

Action Items: Intentions and Thoughts

Sculpting Dreams in the City That Never Sleeps

Darlings, welcome to the city that never sleeps-Manhattan, a place where dreams are born, and ambition flows like the city's iconic skyline. In this chapter, we'll delve into the art of "Sculpting Dreams in the City That Never Sleeps." Here, the streets themselves become a canvas for your aspirations, and every step you take is a brushstroke in your masterpiece. From fitness to life itself, let's explore how Manhattan's relentless energy can inspire you to carve your dreams with passion and purpose.

➢ **A City of Unending Inspiration**: Manhattan's streets are filled with stories of ambition, resilience, and success. It's a place where the very air you breathe is infused with the spirit of dreams realized against all odds.

➢ **The Beat of Manhattan**: Just like the rhythm of a pulsating city, your fitness journey becomes a dance of determination. It's about moving to the beat of your own ambitions as you sculpt both your body and your dreams.

➢ **Every Corner a Story**: Every corner of Manhattan tells a story, from the grandeur of Times Square to the tranquility of the High Line. Your journey is no different, and each milestone becomes a chapter in your narrative.

➢ **The City's Muse**: Manhattan isn't just a backdrop; it's a muse that ignites your creative spirit. Whether you're running along the Hudson River or practicing yoga in Central Park, the city's energy infuses your journey with inspiration.

➢ **Challenges as Opportunities**: In Manhattan, every challenge is an opportunity waiting to be seized. Just as you conquer the hills of Central Park, you conquer life's obstacles with grace, turning them into stepping stones toward your dreams.

➢ **The Art of Hustle**: Manhattan's relentless hustle is your ally in sculpting dreams. It teaches you the value of tenacity, resilience, and the pursuit of excellence, traits that define both your fitness journey and your path to success.

➢ **Diversity of Dreams**: The diversity of Manhattan's neighborhoods mirrors the diversity of dreams you can pursue. Just as you explore different fitness routines, you can explore different facets of your own potential in this vibrant city.

➢ **Sculpting Your Legacy**: Just as the city's landmarks stand as legacies of ambition, your journey through Manhattan is your legacy in the making. It's about leaving your mark on this dynamic city and making your dreams a part of its storied history.

➢ **A Tapestry of Ambition**: In Manhattan, every street corner and skyscraper whispers tales of resilience and triumph. Here, the very air you breathe is filled with the spirit of dreams turned into reality against all odds.

➢ **Moving to the City's Pulse**: Just as the city beats with relentless energy, your fitness journey becomes a dance of purpose and drive. It's about moving in sync with the rhythm of your own ambitions as you sculpt both body and dreams alike.

➢ **Every Landmark, a Legacy**: Each corner of Manhattan holds a story—from the glimmer of Times Square to the calm of High Line.

In the heart of Manhattan, where ambition is the currency, and dreams are the skyline, your journey is an expression of your unique narrative. Let the city's relentless spirit guide you, my darlings, as you sculpt your dreams with passion, determination, and the knowledge that in the city that never sleeps, your aspirations are destined to shine as brightly as the lights of Times Square.

Completed Tasks: Sculpting Dreams Activities

Inspirational Quote

EVER TRIED. EVER FAILED. NO MATTER. TRY AGAIN. FAIL AGAIN. FAIL BETTER. — Samuel Beckett

Action Items: Intentions and Thoughts

Action Items: Intentions and Thoughts

2

Green Lawn Lunges:
Toning Thighs with Every Sunset View

Manhattan, a city that doesn't merely shimmer against the Hudson—it pulsates, a vibrant tapestry woven with tales of ambition, determination, and a dash of unexpected elegance. Here, where time ticks a tad faster, it's not just about chasing the hours, but how you chase them—with a grace that defies gravity and a zest that redefines zeal.

Now imagine: You're venturing through the lush greens of Central Park, and while the city's skyscrapers outline the horizon, eyes are riveted to you. Not because of the shimmer in your jewelry but the strength in your stance. That, my darling, is the Green Lawn Glamour, an art form that transforms every lunge into a poetic dance, marrying fitness with finesse.

In this radiant chapter of The Manhattan Diaries, we'll delve into the artistry behind those Green Lawn Lunges. From the poised descent that carves the silhouette to the exhilarating rise that captures the last rays of the setting sun, you'll unlock the alchemy of turning every move into a mesmerizing spectacle.

But don't be mistaken. This isn't solely a dance of the limbs. It's an ode to the city's soul, about lunging forward with purpose, with passion. It's about finding balance amidst the city's ceaseless rhythm, embracing both the vast open spaces and the intimate nooks they nestle.

So, come along, and let's synchronize our steps with the city's heartbeat. Let's craft a routine that doesn't just sculpt our form but also paints a story on Manhattan's vast canvas. Because, sweetheart, in this city, every lunge is a leap into a new narrative. Ready those legs and set your sights on the horizon, for the city is your stage and the spotlight's on you. Welcome to The Manhattan Diaries—where your grace can mirror the elegance of the city's most iconic scenes.

The Green Lawn Glamour: Elevate Your Fitness Routine

Darlings, welcome to the glamorous world of "The Green Lawn Glamour: Elevate Your Fitness Routine." In the heart of Manhattan, where ambition and elegance entwine, we'll explore how fitness transcends the ordinary. Picture yourself amidst the lush greens of Central Park, where every move transforms into a graceful spectacle. It's not just about toning your body; it's about adding finesse to your every stride. Join me as we delve into the art of elevating your fitness routine to new heights, where every step becomes a dance and every lunge becomes an ode to the city's timeless allure.

➢ **The Green Lawn Glamour Unveiled**: Discover the secrets of the Green Lawn Glamour, where fitness transcends the ordinary and elegance becomes the norm. It's about sculpting your body with grace and finesse.

➢ **Central Park: The Backdrop of Dreams**: Central Park isn't just a park; it's a canvas for your aspirations. Embrace the lush surroundings and let the city's energy inspire your fitness journey.

➢ **The Poetic Dance of Fitness**: Transform your routine into a poetic dance, where every move becomes a mesmerizing spectacle. The Green Lawn Glamour is about capturing the essence of Manhattan's vivacious spirit.

➢ **Sculpting Dreams with Every Lunge**: The Green Lawn Glamour isn't just about toning your body; it's about sculpting your dreams with every lunge. Each graceful move becomes a step toward realizing your aspirations, much like the city's landmarks that symbolize ambition.

➢ **A Symphony of Strength and Elegance**: Your fitness routine becomes a symphony of strength and elegance, where each movement is a note in a melody that celebrates your grace and power. Just as Manhattan's skyline is a testament to human ingenuity, your routine showcases your potential.

➢ **Central Park: Your Fitness Sanctuary**: Central Park offers more than just lush greenery; it's your fitness sanctuary in the heart of the city. Amidst its tranquil landscapes, you find the inspiration to elevate your routine and add finesse to every workout.

➢ **The Art of Balance**: The Green Lawn Glamour teaches you the art of balance, not just in fitness but in life itself. It's about finding equilibrium amidst the city's ceaseless rhythm, much like the harmony between Central Park's natural beauty and Manhattan's urban energy.

➢ **A Dance of Passion and Purpose**: Your fitness journey in Manhattan becomes a dance of passion and purpose. Each step you take is a testament to your determination and a celebration of your own unique narrative, much like the stories etched in the city's iconic landmarks.

➢ **Elegance in Every Stretch**: Embrace the art of stretching as a moment of elegance and mindfulness. Each reach and pose in the Green Lawn Glamour becomes a graceful expression, much like Manhattan's blend of beauty and power—a reminder that fitness can be as refined as it is invigorating.

➢ **The City's Applause**: Each jog and pose in Manhattan's open air feels embraced by the city, its skyline silently cheering you on.

In the heart of Manhattan, where dreams are as tall as skyscrapers and landmarks are symbols of relentless ambition, the Green Lawn Glamour elevates your fitness routine to a new level of grace and elegance. Embrace it, my darlings, and let it be a reflection of your own aspirations in this glamorous city.

Completed Tasks: Green Lawn Glamour Activities

Inspirational Quote

PROBLEMS ARE NOT STOP SIGNS; THEY ARE GUIDELINES. — Robert H. Schuller

Action Items: Intentions and Thoughts

Central Park: Your Urban Oasis for Fitness and Finesse

Darlings, in the heart of bustling Manhattan lies a hidden gem, a sanctuary of lush greenery and tranquility-Central Park. This urban oasis serves as the backdrop for your fitness journey, where you'll discover "Central Park: Your Urban Oasis for Fitness and Finesse." Picture yourself amidst its scenic beauty, where fitness transcends the ordinary, and each move is a brushstroke in your masterpiece. Join me as we explore how this extraordinary park becomes the canvas for sculpting not only your body but also your narrative—a story of ambition, grace, and endless finesse.

- ➤ **Central Park Unveiled**: Let's uncover the enchanting allure of Central Park, where the city's heartbeat merges with nature's serenity, creating the perfect setting for your fitness journey.

- ➤ **Nature's Gym**: Central Park becomes your ultimate fitness playground, offering endless possibilities for outdoor workouts, whether it's running along the reservoir, practicing yoga by the lake, or engaging in bodyweight exercises amidst its green expanse.

- ➤ **Finesse in Fitness**: In Central Park, fitness is not just about strength; it's about finesse. Embrace the gracefulness of your surroundings and elevate your fitness routine to a higher level.

- ➤ **The Reservoir Rendezvous**: Central Park's iconic reservoir becomes your fitness rendezvous, where you can jog along the water's edge, mirroring the elegance of the park's reflective beauty.

- ➤ **Yoga by the Lake**: Find your inner zen as you practice yoga by the picturesque lake. Central Park provides the perfect backdrop for your yoga flow, where fitness seamlessly merges with tranquility.

- ➤ **Balancing Act**: Central Park teaches you the art of balance, not just in your fitness routine but in life itself. It's a reminder that amidst the city's hustle and bustle, there's always a place to find equilibrium.

- ➢ **Elevating Your Routine**: In Central Park, your fitness routine is elevated to an art form. Each workout becomes a masterpiece, much like the city's skyline that symbolizes human achievement.

- ➢ **An Oasis of Inspiration**: Central Park is more than just a place to exercise; it's a source of inspiration. Just as the city's landmarks inspire greatness, the park inspires you to elevate your life, finding finesse in every aspect.

- ➢ **Strength in the Open Air**: Let Central Park's vast landscapes invigorate your strength workouts. From park benches for tricep dips to open fields for lunges, every corner offers a chance to blend power with natural beauty.

- ➢ **The Path Less Traveled**: Embrace the park's winding paths and hidden trails as your running track, where every step immerses you in Central Park's charm, adding an element of adventure to your fitness journey.

- ➢ **Meditation Among the Trees**: Discover the peace of mindfulness practice under Central Park's ancient trees. Each meditation session grounds you, creating a balance between the city's dynamic energy and the park's quiet calm.

- ➢ **Sunrise Sessions**: Begin your day with energizing sunrise workouts in Central Park, letting the first light inspire confidence and set a graceful tone for the day.

In the heart of Manhattan, where ambition meets elegance and dreams are as grand as the city's towering skyscrapers, Central Park serves as your urban oasis. Embrace it, my darlings, and let it be a reflection of your aspirations in this vibrant city. It's where fitness and finesse converge, and every workout is a testament to your ambition and grace amidst the iconic scenes of Manhattan.

Completed Tasks: Fitness and Finesse Activities

Inspirational Quote

WITH THE NEW DAY COMES NEW STRENGTH AND NEW THOUGHTS. —
Eleanor Roosevelt

Action Items: Intentions and Thoughts

Sunset Lunges: Capturing the Essence of Manhattan

Darlings, as the sun sets over the mesmerizing skyline of Manhattan, a unique fitness ritual unfolds-Sunset Lunges. In this radiant chapter, we'll explore the art of "Sunset Lunges: Capturing the Essence of Manhattan." Picture yourself against the backdrop of the city's iconic landmarks, where each lunge becomes a poetic expression of your ambition and grace. It's not just about fitness; it's about capturing the very essence of this vibrant city with every stride you take.

> ➢ **Dancing with the Setting Sun**: Sunset Lunges transform your workout into a dance with the setting sun. Each descent and rise captures the essence of Manhattan's vivacious spirit, just as the city itself transforms as day turns to night.

> ➢ **A City of Endless Inspiration**: Manhattan, with its dazzling lights and towering skyscrapers, serves as your muse. It inspires you to elevate your fitness routine and infuse it with elegance and purpose.

> ➢ **Balance Amidst the Rhythm**: Finding balance amidst the ceaseless rhythm of the city is a skill, much like the art of Sunset Lunges. It's about embracing both the vast open spaces and the intimate corners where you can sculpt not just your body but your narrative.

> ➢ **The City's Ever-Changing Canvas**: Manhattan's skyline is an ever-changing canvas, much like the dynamic nature of Sunset Lunges. With each lunge, you become a part of the city's breathtaking transformation from day to night.

> ➢ **Elegance Amidst the Energy**: Sunset Lunges add a touch of elegance to your fitness routine, mirroring the sophistication of Manhattan's cultural and artistic scene. It's about finding finesse amidst the city's vibrant energy.

➢ **Setting Sun, Rising Ambition**: As the sun sets over Manhattan, your ambition rises. Sunset Lunges become a metaphor for reaching new heights and achieving your dreams, much like the city's towering skyscrapers.

➢ **The Intimate Connection**: Just as you feel an intimate connection with the city during Sunset Lunges, the city itself becomes a part of your journey. You're not just exercising; you're immersing yourself in the very essence of Manhattan.

➢ **A Mesmerizing Spectacle**: Sunset Lunges turn your fitness routine into a mesmerizing spectacle, much like the city's iconic landmarks that draw people from all over the world. Your lunges become a testament to your dedication, ambition, and the allure of Manhattan itself.

➢ **Sunset Reflections**: Each lunge becomes a moment of reflection, as the golden hour envelops you in Manhattan's glow. It's not just exercise—it's time to connect deeply with your goals and let the city's inspiration fuel your journey forward.

➢ **Skyline Silhouettes**: As your form casts a shadow against the fading light, you become part of the city's skyline. Sunset Lunges blend you with Manhattan's silhouette, making your ambition and movement as timeless as the city itself.

In the heart of Manhattan, where dreams are as luminous as the city's lights and landmarks symbolize boundless ambition, Sunset Lunges offer a unique way to capture the essence of this remarkable city. Embrace them, my darlings, and let your every lunge become a graceful brushstroke in the ever-evolving masterpiece of Manhattan's skyline- a skyline that stands tall as a testament to the dreams of those who dared to chase them amidst the breathtaking Manhattan sunset.

Completed Tasks: Sunset Lunges Activities

Inspirational Quote

FAILURE WILL NEVER OVERTAKE ME IF MY DETERMINATION TO SUCCEED IS STRONG ENOUGH. — Og Mandino

GREEN LAWN LUNGES

Action Items: Intentions and Thoughts

The City as Your Stage: Fitness, Finesse, and the Spotlight

Darlings, in the heart of Manhattan, where the city's energy flows like an electric current, you'll discover that every corner, every street, becomes a stage —a stage for fitness, finesse, and the spotlight. Join me as we explore "The City as Your Stage: Fitness, Finesse, and the Spotlight." Picture yourself amidst the dazzling lights of Times Square, where your fitness journey takes center stage, and every move becomes a captivating performance. It's not just about staying in shape; it's about embracing the city's vivacious spirit and letting your grace and ambition shine like a Broadway star.

➢ **Times Square Tango**: In the heart of Times Square, your fitness routine becomes a Tango with the city's vibrant energy. Each step is a dance, and every move is an expression of your grace and determination.

➢ **Iconic Landmarks as Props**: Manhattan's iconic landmarks, from the Statue of Liberty to the Empire State Building, become the props in your fitness performance. They inspire you to reach new heights and elevate your routine.

➢ **The Art of Presentation**: Just as Broadway shows are a spectacle, your fitness journey becomes a performance art. It's about presenting your best self to the world, with the city as your backdrop.

➢ **Choreographing Your Fitness Routine**: Just as a Broadway choreographer crafts a dance; you choreograph your fitness routine. Each movement is a step in your performance, and every workout is a chance to refine your routine.

➢ **Sculpting Dreams Amidst the Skylines**: In the midst of Manhattan's towering skyscrapers, you sculpt not only your body but also your dreams. Your fitness journey becomes a reflection of your ambition, much like the city's iconic skyline.

➢ **Audience of Ambition**: Manhattan becomes your audience of ambition. The city's relentless energy and vibrant spirit inspire you to push your limits and embrace your own spotlight.

➢ **Creating Your Spectacle**: Your fitness journey is not just about exercise; it's about creating a spectacle. Just as Broadway dazzles with its performances, you dazzle with your dedication, turning every workout into a showstopper.

➢ **The Legacy of Your Performance**: Just as the city's landmarks leave a lasting legacy, your fitness journey is your own legacy in the making. It's about leaving your mark on this dynamic city and making your dreams a part of its storied history.

➢ **The Rhythm of the City**: Your workout syncs with Manhattan's pulse, each step echoing the city's rhythm. From the bustling streets to the quieter corners, every part of the city becomes a beat in your unique fitness symphony.

➢ **Lights, Camera, Action**: As the city lights up, your workout gains an extra spark. Whether you're sprinting through Central Park or doing yoga by the Hudson, every movement is a cinematic moment in Manhattan's grand production—starring you.

In the heart of Manhattan, where ambition takes center stage, and dreams are as bright as Broadway lights, your fitness routine becomes a captivating performance. Embrace it, my darlings, and let every move be a testament to your grace, determination, and the allure of Manhattan itself. In this city, you are the star of your own show, and the world is your stage. Welcome to The Manhattan Diaries, where fitness, finesse, and the spotlight converge in the heart of the Big Apple.

CENTRAL PARK'S FITNESS HACKS

Completed Tasks: Your City Stage Activities

Action Items: Intentions and Thoughts

Action Items: Intentions and Thoughts

3

Reservoir Runs: Jogging Tips from Manhattan's Marathoners

Manhattan, a city that doesn't just sleep beneath the blanket of stars—it dreams, dreams so vivid, they spill onto its streets, coursing through every artery, every lane, every byway. And in this city of unbridled aspirations, it isn't just about the destination, but the journey—with elegance, endurance, and electric energy.

Now picture this: You're dashing alongside the Central Park Reservoir, and though the skyline kisses the heavens, onlookers are drawn to you. Not by the brand of your sneakers, but the rhythm of your resolve. That, my love, is the Reservoir Rhapsody, an art form that fuses the grace of a gazelle with the grit of a gladiator.

In this invigorating chapter of The Manhattan Diaries, we'll weave through the wisdom of the city's elite marathoners. From the buoyant bounce that feels like floating on air to the focused sprint that closes the distance between dream and reality, you'll learn the secrets to jog with both joy and judgment.

Yet, this isn't merely a tutorial on technique. It's about imbibing the spirit of Manhattan, jogging not just with speed, but a saga, a sentiment, a song. It's about harmonizing with the heartbeat of the borough, syncing with both its radiant rises and reflective respites.

So, lace up, and let's embark on a journey, not of miles, but of moments, memories, and might. Let's craft a cadence that doesn't just set our pace but sets the pulse of the park. For in Manhattan, every stride, every sprint, every stretch is a story waiting to be scripted. Tighten that ponytail, set your playlist, and remember, the city's rhythm awaits your lead. Welcome to The Manhattan Diaries—where your run can be as riveting as the city's most entrancing rhapsody.

Reservoir Rhapsody: Jogging with Grace and Grit

Darlings, welcome to the sensational world of "Reservoir Rhapsody: Jogging with Grace and Grit." In the heart of Manhattan, where dreams weave seamlessly with the city's rhythm, we'll explore the art of jogging along Central Park's Reservoir. Picture yourself in this urban oasis, where each stride becomes a note in a symphony of elegance and determination. It's not just about jogging; it's about embodying the grace of a gazelle and the grit of a gladiator. Join me as we unravel the secrets of jogging with both poise and power, turning each run into a captivating performance.

> ➤ **The Reservoir Unveiled**: Oh, darlings, Central Park's Reservoir isn't just a body of water; it's a symphony of nature amidst the city's hustle. The energy of Manhattan merges with the serenity of this oasis, creating the perfect backdrop for your jogging journey.

> ➤ **Jogging with Elegance**: In this chapter, we'll explore how jogging is more than just a workout; it's an art form. Learn to infuse every step with elegance, mirroring the sophistication of Manhattan's cultural scene.

> ➤ **Jogging with Elegance**: Now, let's talk about jogging, but not just any jogging—a performance, an art form! It's about infusing every step with elegance, mirroring the sophistication of Manhattan's cultural scene. Imagine jogging as if you're dancing through the city's streets.

> ➤ **Grit and Grace**: Embrace the duality, my loves. It's not just about pushing your limits; it's about doing it with poise and grace. Think of Manhattan's relentless energy, juxtaposed with moments of serene reflection in Central Park. That's the essence we're chasing here.

> ➤ **Rhythm of Central Park**: Picture yourself jogging to the rhythm of Central Park, where every stride is a note in the symphony of the

city's vibrant heartbeat. It's not just about the exercise; it's about becoming one with the park's natural elegance.

➢ **The Runner's Poise**: Let's explore the art of maintaining poise while pushing your limits, akin to a socialite navigating Manhattan's high-society parties with grace. It's about jogging like you own the streets, my loves!

➢ **Duality of Manhattan**: In Manhattan, we embrace duality-the relentless energy of the city juxtaposed with serene moments in Central Park. Jogging becomes a reflection of this dynamic, where you find balance amidst the urban hustle.

➢ **Theatrical Fitness**: Think of jogging as a theatrical performance, my darlings. You are both the star and the audience, and the city's iconic scenes are your backdrop. Each jog is a scene, and every scene tells a story.

➢ **Leaving Your Imprint**: Just as Manhattan's landmarks leave an imprint on the city, your jogging journey becomes your own legacy. It's about leaving your mark, not just on the pavement but on the narrative of this remarkable city.

As we conclude this chapter, darlings, remember that every stride you take in Manhattan is part of a grand performance, just like the city's iconic landmarks. Your jogging journey becomes a testament to your aspirations. It's a reminder that in this city, you are the star of your own show, and every run is a chance to shine amidst the vibrant energy of Manhattan's iconic scenes. So, let the Reservoir Rhapsody be your anthem, where fitness meets finesse, and every performance is a tribute to the city that never sleeps. Welcome to The Manhattan Diaries, where you jog with the grace of a gazelle and the grit of a gladiator, leaving your mark on the storied history of this remarkable city.

Completed Tasks: Jogging with Grace Activities

_____

_____

_____

_____

_____

_____

_____

_____

_____

_____

_____

_____

_____

_____

_____

_____

_____

_____

_____

_____

_____

_____

_____

_____

_____

_____

_____

_____

_____

_____

Inspirational Quote

CHANGE YOUR LIFE TODAY. DON'T GAMBLE ON THE FUTURE. ACT NOW, WITHOUT DELAY. — Simone de Beauvoir

Action Items: Intentions and Thoughts

CENTRAL PARK'S FITNESS HACKS

Central Park Chronicles: Tales from Marathoners

Darlings, welcome to a captivating journey through Central Park in "Central Park Chronicles: Tales from Marathoners." In the heart of Manhattan, where every street holds a story, we'll unveil the wisdom of the city's elite marathoners. Picture yourself amidst the lush greenery of Central Park, where the secrets to endurance and ambition are revealed by those who have conquered the city's marathon trails. Join me as we dive into their tales, exploring how running becomes not just a physical feat but an art form—an expression of grace, ambition, and boundless energy.

- ➤ **The Marathoner's Perspective**: Imagine sipping cocktails with the city's marathon legends, darlings. Hear how they view Central Park as a playground for sculpting not just their endurance but their ambition and grace, darling.

- ➤ **Beneath the Manhattan Skyline**: Think of it, my loves—racing beneath the iconic Manhattan skyline. These marathoners have tales as varied and glamorous as the city's towering skyscrapers. It's a thrilling journey, believe me.

- ➤ **Training Like a New Yorker**: Let's spill the tea on their unique training methods. These marathoners tackle the city like true New Yorkers, and you'll be astonished by their secrets to enduring and thriving in this dynamic metropolis.

- ➤ **Rendezvous in Central Park**: Picture this, my darlings-brunching with these marathon legends amidst the lush beauty of Central Park. Learn how this urban oasis isn't just a backdrop; it's their training sanctuary, where ambition and nature mingle like old friends.

- ➤ **New York's Marathon Culture**: Now, let's spill the juicy details about New York's marathon culture. These runners aren't just athletes; they're part of a vibrant community that thrives on the city's electric energy. It's like being part of the most exclusive social club, but with sneakers and sweatbands.

➢ **From Struggles to Triumphs**: Prepare to be moved, my loves, as you listen to the tales of marathoners who've conquered not only the streets but also their own personal struggles. Their stories of resilience are as captivating as a Broadway drama, and just as inspiring.

➢ **Central Park**: Their Running Muse: Explore how Central Park inspires these marathoners to push their limits and achieve their dreams. It's a love story between the runners and this green heart of Manhattan.

➢ **Lessons from the Finish Line**: Discover the life lessons these marathoners have learned from crossing the finish line in the greatest city in the world. Their wisdom goes beyond running, my darlings; it's about conquering life's marathons with style and substance.

➢ **Rhythm of the Park**: Discover how each runner finds a unique rhythm in Central Park's winding paths. For them, every incline, curve, and descent holds a familiar beat, blending their own pulse with the heartbeat of the city itself.

➢ **Fueling the Dream**: Learn the rituals and favorite refueling spots of these elite marathoners, from post-run smoothies to hidden cafes. These places not only nourish their bodies but also serve as havens of inspiration and camaraderie in the marathon journey.

In the heart of Manhattan, where ambition flows like champagne and dreams reach skyscraper heights, Central Park becomes the backdrop for tales of grace, ambition, and boundless energy. Embrace it, my darlings, and let these marathoners' stories be the inspiration for your own narrative in The Manhattan Diaries.

Completed Tasks: Tales and Chronicles Activities

Inspirational Quote

LIFE APPEARS TO ME TOO SHORT TO BE SPENT IN NURSING ANIMOSITY OR REGISTERING WRONGS. — Charlotte Bronte

Action Items: Intentions and Thoughts

Running with Heart: Syncing with Manhattan's Spirit

Darlings, in the heart of Manhattan, where the city's spirit pulses like a heartbeat, we'll explore "Running with Heart: Syncing with Manhattan's Spirit." Picture yourself amidst the vibrant streets, where every step becomes a dance to the rhythm of the city. It's not just about running; it's about syncing with Manhattan's soul, embracing its relentless energy, and finding your own heartbeat within the city's grandeur. Join me as we dive into this exhilarating chapter, where running is more than a workout—it's a passionate embrace of the city's spirit.

> ➢ **Manhattan's Electric Pulse**: Imagine running in a city where the pulse of Manhattan itself propels you forward. Each stride syncs with the vibrant energy that courses through every street and skyscraper.

> ➢ **The Run as a Symphony**: Let's envision running as a symphony, my darlings. Your steps are the notes, and the city's sights and sounds compose the music. It's about becoming one with the urban melody.

> ➢ **Finding Serenity Amidst Chaos**: Just like Central Park offers moments of serenity amidst the bustling city; your run becomes a journey of balance—embracing both the chaos and tranquility that Manhattan offers.

> ➢ **Running as a Love Affair**: Envision your run as a passionate love affair with Manhattan. Each step is a declaration of your adoration for the city's soul, and every street becomes a secret rendezvous with its vibrant spirit.

> ➢ **The Runway of Fifth Avenue**: Think of your run along Fifth Avenue as a runway show, my loves. You're not just running; you're

strutting your stuff amidst the city's fashionable elegance, turning every block into a chic catwalk.

➢ **The Manhattan Marathon**: Explore the thrill of training for the New York City Marathon, where running becomes a marathon of emotions, challenges, and triumphs. It's like starring in your own epic drama right on the city's stage.

➢ **Sunset Runs on the Hudson**: Imagine running along the Hudson River at sunset, where the city's shimmering lights come to life. It's a moment of pure magic, and your run becomes a poetic dance with the city's skyline.

➢ **Running into the Future**: Just as Manhattan constantly reinvents itself; your runs represent your journey into the future. Each step is a stride towards your aspirations, much like the city's continuous evolution.

➢ **The Bridges of Manhattan**: Envision your runs taking you across the iconic bridges of Manhattan, each step a passage over history and into the heart of the city. As you rise above the river, your cadence matches the strength and resilience of these architectural marvels.

➢ **The City Lights Finale**: Picture yourself finishing a night run through Manhattan's dazzling streets, where every glowing light feels like an audience cheering you on. The city's nighttime sparkle reflects your determination, turning your journey into a radiant celebration of ambition and grit.

In the heart of Manhattan, where dreams are woven into the very fabric of the city, running with heart becomes an expression of love, ambition, and unyielding spirit. Embrace it, my darlings, and let your runs echo the elegance of Manhattan's most iconic scenes in The Manhattan Diaries.

Completed Tasks: Running with Heart Activities

_____
_____
_____
_____
_____
_____
_____
_____
_____
_____
_____
_____
_____
_____
_____
_____
_____
_____
_____
_____
_____
_____
_____
_____
_____
_____
_____

Inspirational Quote

THE SHOE THAT FITS ONE PERSON PINCHES ANOTHER. THERE IS NO RECIPE FOR LIVING THAT SUITS ALL CASES. — Carl Jung

Action Items: Intentions and Thoughts

The Pulse of the Park: Crafting Your Cadence

Darlings, running through Central Park is more than exercise—it's a creative journey. "The Pulse of the Park: Crafting Your Cadence" invites you to turn each stride into a melody, blending the city's energy with the park's natural beauty. From the peaceful Ramble at dawn to the graceful Reservoir, every path inspires a unique rhythm. Whether you're moving with the city's pulse or finding calm in nature, your run becomes an elegant dance, a personal expression in the heart of Manhattan.

➤ **Central Park's Melodic Muse**: Imagine Central Park as your muse, darlings. With each step, you're composing a melody that harmonizes with the park's beauty, turning your run into a symphony of nature and ambition.

➤ **Running with Elegance**: Let's envision running as a graceful dance, my loves. Your cadence is your choreography, and the park's winding paths are your stage. It's about exuding elegance amidst the city's chaos.

➤ **Finding Your Tempo**: Just as the city's streets have varying tempos, your run allows you to find your own rhythm. Whether it's the fast-paced beat of Midtown or the tranquil melody of Central Park, you craft your cadence to match the moment.

➤ **Dawn Serenades in the Ramble**: Envision your run at dawn in the Ramble, where the park's melodies are at their most enchanting. It's a moment of serenity amidst the city's daily crescendo, and your cadence becomes a harmonious serenade.

➤ **The Reservoir Waltz:** Picture your run along the Reservoir's edge as a waltz, my loves. You glide along the water's edge, mirroring the elegance of Manhattan's Upper East Side. It's a dance of sophistication and style.

➢ **The Pulse of the Parkrun**: Explore the vibrant parkrun community, where your cadence becomes part of a larger, rhythmic tapestry. You're not just running; you're participating in a shared dance with fellow park enthusiasts.

➢ **Bridge Rhythms**: Imagine conquering the bridges within Central Park, where your cadence matches the city's ebb and flow. It's like crossing into different chapters of your run, each with its own unique tempo.

➢ **Central Park as Your Muse**: Just as artists find inspiration in Central Park's beauty, your runs become your creative expression. Your cadence is your brushstroke on the canvas of Manhattan's landscape, crafting your unique masterpiece.

➢ **Sunset Sprints at the Bow Bridge**: Imagine the beauty of ending your run at the Bow Bridge as the sun dips below the skyline. With each step, your cadence mirrors the golden glow, making your run a poetic journey through Manhattan's most serene hours.

➢ **Harmony of Hustle and Calm**: Picture your strides capturing the city's dual energy—its relentless hustle and serene calm. Running through Central Park's tranquil paths against the city's vibrant backdrop, you find harmony, a unique cadence that syncs ambition with inner peace.

In the heart of Manhattan, where every moment is a story waiting to be told, crafting your cadence in Central Park becomes an art form—an expression of your elegance, ambition, and boundless spirit. Embrace it, my darlings, and let your runs echo the grace of Manhattan's most iconic scenes in The Manhattan Diaries.

Completed Tasks: Crafting Your Candence Activities

Inspirational Quote

THE INDISPENSABLE FIRST STEP TO GETTING THE THINGS YOU WANT OUT OF LIFE IS THIS: DECIDE WHAT YOU WANT. —— Ben Stein

Action Items: Intentions and Thoughts

Music, Miles, and Manhattan: Your Running Playlist

Darlings, welcome to "Music, Miles, and Manhattan: Your Running Playlist." In the heart of Manhattan, where every street has a soundtrack, we'll explore the art of curating the perfect running playlist for your city escapades. Picture yourself on the vibrant streets, where every step becomes a dance to the rhythm of your chosen tunes. It's not just about running; it's about syncing your soul with the city's heartbeat and letting your playlist be the backdrop to your urban adventures. Join me as we dive into this electrifying chapter, where music isn't just a companion-it's the soundtrack to your Manhattan story.

> ➤ **The Soundtrack of the City**: Imagine the city's bustling streets as a stage, and your running playlist as the soundtrack. Each song sets the mood for your journey, turning the streets into a dynamic dance floor.

> ➤ **Energetic Anthems for Midtown**: Let's talk about the energetic anthems that keep you going through Midtown's fast-paced streets. It's like having your personal DJ fueling your run amidst the skyscrapers.

> ➤ **Soulful Tunes in Central Park**: Envision running in Central Park to soulful tunes that match the park's tranquility. It's a moment of serenity amidst the city's daily crescendo, and your playlist becomes the backdrop to your own private concert.

> ➤ **Sunset Serenades along the Hudson**: Picture yourself running along the Hudson River at sunset, with your playlist as the backdrop to the city's shimmering lights. It's like a private concert amidst the most breathtaking views.

➢ **Broadway Beats**: Let's explore the lively beats of Broadway tunes in your playlist. It's as if you're performing in your very own Broadway show, with the city's iconic theaters as your stage.

➢ **Empire State of Mind**: Envision conquering the city's streets with "Empire State of Mind" as your anthem. It's not just a song; it's a declaration of your love affair with Manhattan.

➢ **Jazz and Jazzercise**: Think of incorporating jazzy tunes into your playlist for a bit of jazzercise flair. It's like merging the sophistication of Manhattan's jazz scene with the high-energy pulse of your run.

➢ **The Park's Natural Harmony**: Imagine running in Central Park to acoustic tunes that match the park's natural harmony. It's a serene escape, where your playlist becomes the perfect complement to the park's beauty.

➢ **Classic Rock on the Brooklyn Bridge**: Picture crossing the Brooklyn Bridge with classic rock tunes as your backdrop. The powerful guitar riffs mirror the iconic structure's strength, turning your run into a rock-and-roll journey over the East River and into the heart of Manhattan.

➢ **Downtown Disco**: Imagine running through the vibrant streets of SoHo and the Lower East Side with upbeat disco tracks fueling your pace. Each step becomes a groove as the neighborhood's eclectic vibe aligns with the danceable beats, adding flair to every mile.

In the heart of Manhattan, where every street is a stage and every moment a scene, your running playlist becomes the soundtrack to your urban escapades. Embrace it, my darlings, and let your runs echo the stylish charm of Manhattan's most iconic scenes in The Manhattan Diaries.

Completed Tasks: Running Playlist Activities

Inspirational Quote

I DID NOT DIRECT MY LIFE. I DIDN'T DESIGN IT. I NEVER MADE DECISIONS. THINGS ALWAYS CAME UP AND MADE THEM FOR ME. THAT'S WHAT LIFE IS. — B. F. Skinner

Action Items: Intentions and Thoughts

Action Items: Intentions and Thoughts

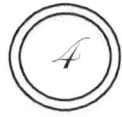

Bow Bridge Ballet:
Poise, Posture, and Plies in the Park

Manhattan, a city that doesn't just admire the lights—it becomes them, illuminating every contour and curvature with tales of passion, precision, and unparalleled poise. And in this city of countless stages, it isn't just about the standing ovations at the end; it's about the rehearsals, the sweat, the swansong—with elegance, élan, and a touch of enigma.

Envision this: You're pirouetting by the iconic Bow Bridge, with the sun's rays painting you gold, and every observer is spellbound, not by the designer of your tutu, but the tapestry of your talent. That, dearest, is the Bow Bridge Ballet, an art form that melds the mystique of moonlit waters with the magic of Manhattan.

In this entrancing chapter of The Manhattan Diaries, we'll delve deep into the dance that defines the city's spirit. From the whispering waltz to the tantalizing tango of a dancer whose heart beats in choreographed cadence, you'll be initiated into the intricacies of making Central Park your personal parquet.

But this is more than mere movement—it's meditation. It's about resonating with the romance of the city, dancing not just with feet but with feelings, fantasies, fervor. It's about the symbiosis with both the glimmers of the Great Lawn and the serenity of the surrounding skyline, embracing the dichotomy of Manhattan's dreams and dramas.

So, slide into those ballet shoes, feel the world fade, and let's float into a fantasy, where every plie, every pas de deux, every pirouette is poetry in motion. Because, darling, in Manhattan, every dance step is a diary entry waiting to be etched. Stretch that leg, point those toes, for the city is your stage, your spotlight. Welcome to The Manhattan Diaries—where your ballet can be as breathtaking as the city's most captivating chorus.

Bow Bridge Ballet: Dancing with Manhattan's Heartbeat

Darlings, it's time to waltz into the enchanting world of "Bow Bridge Ballet: Dancing with Manhattan's Heartbeat." In a city that radiates elegance, precision, and passion, we'll explore the art of ballet, where every graceful movement resonates with Manhattan's soul. Imagine yourself pirouetting by the iconic Bow Bridge, where the sun's rays transform you into pure gold, and the city's observers are spellbound by your talent, not your attire. This is the Bow Bridge Ballet, an exquisite art form that merges the mystique of moonlit waters with the magic of Manhattan. Join me as we delve into this mesmerizing chapter, where ballet isn't just a dance—it's a passionate embrace of the city's spirit.

➢ **Elegance by the Bridge**: Explore how the Bow Bridge Ballet encapsulates the very essence of Manhattan's elegance, where each movement becomes a poetic expression of the city's heartbeat.

➢ **The Iconic Bow Bridge**: Delve into the allure of the iconic Bow Bridge, where every pirouette is a love letter to this exquisite landmark.

➢ **Central Park's Dance Floor**: Discover the secrets of making Central Park your own personal parquet, where lush greenery and the iconic bridge set the stage for your ballet dreams.

➢ **More than Movement, Meditation**: Uncover how ballet transcends mere movement to become a form of meditation, a way of connecting with the city's romance, and an escape into the dreams and dramas of Manhattan.

➢ **Moonlit Whispers by the Water**: Envision dancing under the moonlight, the city's lights reflected in the water below. It's like a secret rendezvous with Manhattan's mystique, where every movement is a whispered promise.

➢ **Manhattan's Ballet of Dreams**: Think of the city as our grand stage, and your ballet as a dance of dreams. Each arabesque is a leap towards your aspirations, mirroring the city's ceaseless pursuit of ambition.

➢ **The Bow Bridge Embrace**: Picture the Bow Bridge as your dance partner, the arches framing your performance. It's like sharing a tender embrace with a symbol of the city's timeless allure.

➢ **Grace amidst the Urban Drama**: Imagine dancing amidst the city's hustle and bustle, finding moments of grace amidst the urban drama. It's like adding a touch of elegance to the city's vibrant tapestry.

➢ **Sunrise Serenade**: Picture yourself dancing at sunrise, the soft morning light casting a golden hue over Bow Bridge. Each movement feels like a quiet celebration of new beginnings, with the city just starting to stir awake, witnessing your graceful dawn performance.

➢ **Reflections of Resilience**: As you dance by the water's edge, the lake reflects not only the skyline but your own strength and dedication. Each graceful leap and poised plié becomes a symbol of Manhattan's resilient spirit, reminding you that every movement is a testament to inner strength.

➢ **Ballet and Skyline Synergy**: Imagine each pirouette framed by Manhattan's skyline, blending artistry with ambition as you dance in harmony with the city's energy and elegance.

In the heart of Manhattan, where every moment is a story waiting to be told, the Bow Bridge Ballet becomes a captivating dance of passion, precision, and poise. Embrace it, my darlings, and let your ballet echo the grace of Manhattan's most iconic scenes in The Manhattan Diaries.

Completed Tasks: Ballet Dancing Activities

Inspirational Quote

I DON'T BELIEVE YOU HAVE TO BE BETTER THAN EVERYBODY ELSE. I BELIEVE YOU HAVE TO BE BETTER THAN YOU EVER THOUGHT YOU COULD BE. — Ken Venturi

Action Items: Intentions and Thoughts

Central Park's Dance Floor: Where Dreams Take Center Stage

Darlings, welcome to "Central Park's Dance Floor: Where Dreams Take Center Stage." In the heart of Manhattan, where dreams are woven into the very fabric of the city, Central Park becomes our enchanting dance floor. Picture yourself amidst the lush greenery, where every step is a graceful move toward your aspirations, and where dreams are not just whispered but danced to life. Join me as we delve into this exhilarating chapter, where Central Park transforms into a grand stage, and where the city's elegance converges with the boundless dreams of its residents.

➢ **The Park's Ballet**: Picture, my darlings, Central Park as our enchanting ballet stage. Every movement becomes an expression of our dreams, a dance of ambition that harmonizes with the park's timeless beauty. It's like crafting a symphony with every step.

➢ **Iconic Landmarks as Backdrops**: Let's talk about how Central Park's iconic landmarks, such as the Bow Bridge and Bethesda Terrace, transform into stunning backdrops for our dance of dreams. Every arabesque is a graceful stroke on the canvas of the city, framed by the arches that echo our elegance.

➢ **Cityscape as Your Audience**: Envision the city's skyscrapers as our audience, their lights twinkling in admiration of our performance. It's as if the entire city pauses to witness our dreams taking center stage, applauding our pursuit of ambition.

➢ **Parkside Serenades**: Envision dancing in the park as the sun sets, serenaded by the sounds of nature. It's like a private performance, where every step is a note in the symphony of Central Park.

➢ **Theatrical Twirls**: Think of your dance as a theatrical production, with Central Park as your grand stage. Each twirl and leap becomes a scene in your own Manhattan drama.

➢ **Dreams in Full Bloom**: Imagine dancing amidst Central Park's blooming flowers, where your aspirations blossom alongside the park's natural beauty. It's a reminder that dreams can thrive in the heart of the city.

➢ **Urban Enchantment**: Explore the enchantment of dancing in an urban oasis. Central Park is not just a park; it's a haven where dreams take flight, and your dance becomes the embodiment of Manhattan's elegance and ambition.

➢ **Sunrise Waltz:** Picture yourself dancing as dawn breaks over Central Park, each step infused with the soft, golden light of sunrise. It's a quiet, intimate moment where your dreams awaken alongside the city.

➢ **Reflections in the Lake:** Imagine the park's serene lake mirroring each movement, doubling the beauty of every pirouette and leap. It's as if Manhattan itself is reflecting your aspirations, amplifying your elegance.

➢ **Elegance Amidst Chaos**: Dancing through the city's hustle adds grace to the urban drama, showing that dreams shine brightest amidst Manhattan's lively rhythm.

➢ **Moonlit Movements:** Envision dancing under a starlit sky, the moonlight casting a gentle glow across Central Park. Your dance becomes a timeless performance, shared only with the park and the quiet magic of Manhattan at night.

In the heart of Manhattan, where dreams are etched into the city's very soul, Central Park's dance floor becomes a stage where our aspirations take center stage. Embrace it, my darlings, and let your dance echo the grace of Manhattan's most iconic scenes in The Manhattan Diaries.

Completed Tasks: City Park Dance Floor Activities

Inspirational Quote

I AM NOT A HAS-BEEN. I AM A WILL BE. — Lauren Bacall

Action Items: Intentions and Thoughts

Elegance in Motion: The Art of Ballet as Meditation

Darlings, welcome to "Elegance in Motion: The Art of Ballet as Meditation." In the heart of Manhattan, where life's rhythm often feels like a bustling symphony, we'll explore how ballet transcends mere movement to become a form of meditation. Imagine yourself in a world of grace and precision, where every plie and arabesque becomes a tranquil escape into the city's romance. Join me as we delve into this captivating chapter, where ballet isn't just dance-it's a soulful connection with the heart of Manhattan.

➢ **Ballet's Serene Flow**: Imagine, darlings, the serenity that ballet brings amidst the bustling city. Each graceful movement becomes a flowing meditation, a dance that harmonizes with the city's own heartbeat. It's as if the chaos of Manhattan fades away, leaving only the elegance of your ballet.

➢ **The Dance of Breathing**: Let's discuss how ballet becomes a dance of breathing, where every inhale and exhale synchronizes with your movements. It's like finding your inner calm in the midst of the city's whirlwind, a moment to pause and reflect amidst the urban symphony.

➢ **Central Park's Tranquil Embrace**: Envision Central Park as your sanctuary, where the lush greenery cradles your ballet with nature's grace. It's like dancing in harmony with Manhattan's serene side, a tranquil escape from the urban hustle.

➢ **Urban Meditation**: Think of ballet as an urban meditation, where every pirouette and plie becomes a moment of reflection, a respite from the city's endless energy. It's your way of finding balance amidst the whirlwind of Manhattan, a graceful pause in the midst of the city's drama.

➤ **Dancing to the City's Rhythm**: Imagine ballet as a dance to the city's rhythm, where each plie and leap follows the pulse of Manhattan. It's as if the city itself becomes your partner in this elegant meditation.

➤ **Twilight Elegance**: Picture dancing in the twilight, with the city's lights twinkling around you. It's like stepping into a dream, where every movement is a brushstroke on the canvas of Manhattan's skyline.

➤ **Ballet's Timeless Appeal**: Let's talk about how ballet transcends time, connecting us with the past and future. It's like an ageless meditation, where the city's history and future aspirations merge in each graceful step.

➤ **Cityscape as Your Stage**: Envision Manhattan's skyscrapers as your stage, their towering presence a reminder of the city's ambition. It's as if the entire city applauds your meditation, appreciating the elegance you bring to its energetic streets.

➤ **Grace in Every Glance:** Picture each movement as a quiet exchange with the city itself, a subtle nod to Manhattan's spirit. Ballet becomes a way to carry grace within, even as the city buzzes around you, turning each glance into a shared moment of calm.

➤ **Harmony in Motion**: Dance to Manhattan's hum, each movement syncing with the city's pulse, creating a serene blend of art and urban rhythm.

In the heart of Manhattan, where every moment is a chance to connect with the city's essence, ballet becomes a mesmerizing meditation that mirrors the elegance and ambition of the city. Embrace it, my darlings, and let your ballet become a serene reflection of Manhattan's most iconic scenes in The Manhattan Diaries.

Completed Tasks: Elegance in Motion Activities

Inspirational Quote

KNOWING IS NOT ENOUGH; WE MUST APPLY. WILLING IS NOT ENOUGH; WE MUST DO. — Johann Wolfgang von Goethe

Action Items: Intentions and Thoughts

Poetry in Motion: Ballet's Intricate Dance with Manhattan's Dichotomy

Darlings, welcome to "Poetry in Motion: Ballet's Intricate Dance with Manhattan's Dichotomy." In the heart of this magnificent city, where contrasts and contradictions are woven into its very fabric, we'll explore how ballet's intricate dance mirrors Manhattan's multifaceted essence. Picture yourself in a world of elegance and precision, where every arabesque and plie becomes a delicate expression of the city's dynamic dichotomy. Join me as we delve into this enthralling chapter, where ballet isn't just dance—it's a poetic interpretation of Manhattan's many faces.

> ➤ **Ballet's Graceful Language**: Let's unravel how ballet becomes a graceful language that speaks to Manhattan's contradictions. Each movement becomes a stanza, expressing the city's dualities with finesse.

> ➤ **Iconic Landmarks as Inspiration**: Delve into how Manhattan's iconic landmarks, like Times Square and the serene Central Park, inspire your ballet's intricate choreography. They are the muses behind every pirouette and plie.

> ➤ **Harmonizing with Chaos and Calm**: Envision your ballet as a harmonious dance that embraces both the city's chaos and its calm. It's like finding balance amidst the vibrant energy and tranquil oases of Manhattan.

> ➤ **Urban Poetry**: Think of ballet as urban poetry, where every leap and twirl creates verses that capture the city's relentless ambition and its serene respites. Your dance becomes a poetic reflection of Manhattan's soul.

> ➤ **Cityscape as Your Canvas**: Imagine the city's bustling streets and towering skyscrapers as your canvas. With each ballet movement,

you paint a vivid picture that captures Manhattan's vibrant spirit and its moments of stillness.

➢ **Dancing Through the Seasons**: Picture your ballet evolving with the seasons, from the vibrant blooms of spring to the cozy elegance of winter. It's like choreographing your dance to the changing moods of Manhattan itself.

➢ **Finding Beauty in Contrast**: Let's explore how ballet allows you to find beauty in the contrast of Manhattan's urban landscape. Your dance becomes a reflection of the city's dichotomy, celebrating its dynamic diversity.

➢ **Ballet's Timeless Appeal**: Envision ballet as a timeless art form, mirroring the enduring spirit of Manhattan. Each movement transcends the present, connecting you with the city's rich history and its limitless future.

➢ **The Symphony of City Lights:** Imagine performing under the city's twinkling lights, where every step in your ballet mirrors Manhattan's sparkle. It's a dance that captures both the glamour and grit of the city, reflecting its constant shimmer.

➢ **Steps Through History:** Envision each ballet movement connecting you with Manhattan's layered past. Dancing here becomes a tribute, paying homage to the city's storied history as you move gracefully through its timeless landmarks.

In the heart of Manhattan, where the city's dichotomy is both its challenge and its allure, ballet becomes a poetic dance that mirrors the complexity and ambition of the city. Embrace it, my darlings, and let your ballet become a lyrical reflection of Manhattan's most iconic scenes in The Manhattan Diaries.

Completed Tasks: Poetry in Motion Activities

Inspirational Quote

LEAP, AND THE NET WILL APPEAR. — John Burroughs

Action Items: Intentions and Thoughts

Action Items: Intentions and Thoughts

5

Sheep Meadow Yoga:
Stretching Amidst the Skyscrapers' Silhouette

Manhattan, a city that doesn't just breathe—it sighs and hums, with every exhale telling tales of aspirations, ambitions, and a touch of ancient wisdom. And in this city, cradled by an orchestra of incessant rhythms, it isn't merely about chasing dreams; it's about grounding them—with grace, grit, and a touch of the ethereal.

Imagine, if you will: You're unfolding your mat on Sheep Meadow, with every gaze instinctively resting on you, not because of the brand of your leggings, but the silhouette of your soul against the majestic Manhattan skyline. That, my dear, is the Sheep Meadow Serenade, a symphony that seamlessly fuses the fluidity of yoga with the fervor of the city.

In this enchanting chapter of The Manhattan Diaries, we'll embark on a journey that's less about the physical and more about the metaphysical. From the tranquil transcendence of the Tree Pose to the audacious ardor of the Warrior, you'll learn to stretch not just your body but your boundaries amidst the city's pulsating heart.

But this isn't merely about poses and postures—far from it. It's about harmonizing with the hum of the city, aligning with an aura that's as timeless as the tale of Manhattan itself. It's about feeling both the openness of the meadow and the embrace of the towering titans around, encapsulating the essence of Manhattan's myriad moods.

So, unroll that mat, inhale the synergy, and let's sculpt stories that are as expansive as the sky above and as profound as the earth below. Because, darling, in Manhattan, every asana is an anthem, a whispered secret between the city and the self. Find your center, feel the cosmos, for the city beckons your breath. Welcome to The Manhattan Diaries—where your yoga can be as mesmerizing as the city's most magical moments.

Yoga in the Heart of Manhattan

Darlings, welcome to "Yoga in the Heart of Manhattan." In the midst of this captivating city, where life's pace often feels like an exhilarating dance, we'll explore the art of yoga as a transformative journey. Picture yourself amidst the towering skyscrapers, where yoga becomes a serene oasis— a moment of stillness amidst the city's endless energy. Join me as we delve into this enthralling chapter, where yoga isn't just exercise; it's a soulful connection with the heart of Manhattan.

➢ **Yoga's Urban Symphony**: Picture yoga as an urban symphony, where each pose is a note in the vibrant melody of the city. It's like dancing to Manhattan's rhythm, where the streets themselves become your dance floor.

➢ **Central Park's Tranquil Haven**: Envision Central Park as your personal sanctuary, where yoga's embrace finds solace amidst the lush greenery. It's a tranquil escape in the heart of the city's bustling drama.

➢ **The Metaphysical Journey**: Let's delve into the metaphysical side of yoga, where it's not just about physical exercise but aligning with Manhattan's timeless essence. It's a spiritual journey that connects you with the city's diverse moods.

➢ **Yoga as an Anthem**: Think of yoga as an anthem, a whispered secret shared between you and the city. Each pose becomes a profound moment of connection with Manhattan's dynamic spirit, a dance of the soul.

➢ **Yoga Amidst Iconic Landmarks**: Imagine practicing yoga amidst Manhattan's iconic landmarks, from Times Square's electric energy to the serenity of Central Park's Bow Bridge. Your poses become a dance with the city's history and future.

➢ **Finding Balance in the Chaos**: Explore how yoga helps you find balance in the midst of Manhattan's whirlwind. It's like a moment of calm within the urban storm, a chance to recharge amidst the city's relentless pace.

➢ **Sunset Yoga**: Capturing Manhattan's Magic Hour: Picture practicing yoga during the city's enchanting sunset hours. It's like becoming part of Manhattan's nightly spectacle, where every pose is a brushstroke on the canvas of the skyline.

➢ **Yoga as Manhattan's Muse**: Let's talk about how Manhattan inspires your yoga practice. It's as if the city itself is your muse, infusing your poses with its energy, ambition, and elegance.

➢ **The Art of Yoga as Self-Discovery**: Envision yoga as a journey of self-discovery amidst the city's diverse tapestry. Each pose becomes a moment of reflection, a way to connect with both the city and your inner self.

➢ **Skyline Sunrise Meditation**: Start your day with a sunrise meditation against the Manhattan skyline, blending inner calm with the city's awakening energy.

➢ **Poses Inspired by the City's Pulse:** Imagine each yoga pose drawing inspiration from Manhattan's dynamic pulse. Whether it's the grounded strength of a warrior pose or the fluid grace of a dancer, your practice mirrors the city's balance of resilience and elegance.

In the heart of Manhattan, where every moment is a chance to connect with the city's essence, yoga becomes a transformative journey that mirrors the complexity and ambition of the city. Embrace it, my darlings, and let your yoga practice become a mesmerizing journey that captures the very soul of Manhattan in The Manhattan Diaries.

Completed Tasks: Yoga Activities

Inspirational Quote

THE FIRST STEP TOWARD SUCCESS IS TAKEN WHEN YOU REFUSE TO BE A CAPTIVE OF THE ENVIRONMENT IN WHICH YOU FIRST FIND YOURSELF. — Mark Caine

Action Items: Intentions and Thoughts

Sheep Meadow's Serenade

Darlings, welcome to "Sheep Meadow's Serenade." In the heart of this bustling city, where dreams rise as high as its skyscrapers, we'll explore the art of yoga amidst the serene oasis of Sheep Meadow. Imagine unrolling your mat amidst Central Park's lush greenery, where every pose becomes a melody, a serenade to the majestic Manhattan skyline. Join me as we delve into this enchanting chapter, where yoga isn't just a practice; it's a symphony that harmonizes with the spirit of Manhattan.

> ➤ **Central Park's Urban Retreat**: Imagine Central Park as your secret urban retreat, where the city's ceaseless energy fades away, and you find solace in the embrace of Sheep Meadow. It's like a whispered serenade to Manhattan's bustling heart.

> ➤ **Yoga's Dance with Nature**: Envision yoga as a graceful dance with nature, your poses synchronized with the park's gentle rhythms. It's a ballet with the breeze, a waltz with the trees, and an ode to the harmony of the meadow.

> ➤ **The Skyline as Your Backdrop**: Picture the Manhattan skyline as the backdrop to your yoga practice— a breathtaking canvas for your poses. It's like painting your silhouette against the city's dreams, a dance that captures its timeless allure.

> ➤ **Sheep Meadow's Timeless Aura**: Explore how Sheep Meadow holds a timeless aura, where yoga becomes a bridge between the city's past, present, and future. It's as if each pose connects you with the rich tapestry of Manhattan's history.

> ➤ **Yoga at Magic Hour**: Picture practicing yoga during Manhattan's enchanting magic hour, as the sun sets behind the skyline. It's like becoming part of the city's nightly spectacle, where each pose is a brushstroke on the canvas of the evening sky.

➢ **Sheep Meadow's Serenity**: Explore how Sheep Meadow's serenity becomes your haven amidst the urban chaos. It's where the city's relentless pace fades away, and you find peace in the heart of Manhattan.

➢ **Yoga as Manhattan's Whisper**: Let's talk about how yoga becomes Manhattan's whisper, a secret shared between you and the city. Each pose is a moment of connection, a silent dialogue with the vibrant spirit of Manhattan.

➢ **Yoga's Cityscape Choreography**: Envision your yoga practice as a choreography with the cityscape. Your poses become elegant movements against the backdrop of Manhattan's iconic landmarks, a dance that mirrors the metropolis.

➢ **Sheep Meadow's Storyteller**: Imagine Sheep Meadow as a storyteller, where each blade of grass and rustle of leaves holds a tale. Your yoga practice becomes a chapter in the epic narrative of Manhattan's ever-evolving story.

➢ **Flowing with Meadow's Melody**: Each yoga flow syncs with the meadow's gentle rhythm, creating a harmony with Manhattan's quiet side.

➢ **Morning Glow and Meadow Dew**: Start your day with sunrise yoga, as the meadow's dewdrops reflect the city's first light. It's a gentle, radiant greeting from Manhattan, infusing your practice with calm and clarity.

In the heart of Manhattan, where the city's energy meets the tranquility of Sheep Meadow, your yoga practice becomes a serenade—a connection with the soul of the city. Embrace it, my darlings, and let your yoga practice become a mesmerizing symphony that captures the essence of Manhattan in The Manhattan Diaries.

Completed Tasks: Yoga Spaces Activities

Inspirational Quote

CONSULT NOT YOUR FEARS BUT YOUR HOPES AND YOUR DREAMS. THINK NOT ABOUT YOUR FRUSTRATIONS, BUT ABOUT YOUR UNFULFILLED POTENTIAL. CONCERN YOURSELF NOT WITH WHAT YOU TRIED AND FAILED IN, BUT WITH WHAT IT IS STILL POSSIBLE FOR YOU TO DO. — Pope John XXIII

Action Items: Intentions and Thoughts

Metaphysical Yoga

Darlings, welcome to "Metaphysical Yoga." In the heart of this vibrant city, where each step feels like a chapter in a dazzling novel, we'll delve into the art of yoga as a metaphysical journey. Picture yourself amidst the iconic Manhattan landmarks, where yoga becomes more than physical exercise—it's a spiritual connection with the timeless essence of the city. Join me as we explore this enchanting chapter, where yoga isn't just about poses; it's about aligning with Manhattan's diverse moods and capturing its enduring spirit.

➢ **The Manhattan Metamorphosis**: Picture yoga as a transformative journey, my darlings, where each pose dances with the city's ever-changing spirit. It's like capturing the essence of Manhattan's relentless evolution, a choreography of ambition and resilience that mirrors your own transformation.

➢ **Yoga as a Spiritual Bridge**: Let's dive into the spiritual side of yoga, where it becomes a bridge between your soul and the city's beating heart. Each pose is a profound connection, like whispering secrets with Manhattan's past, present, and future—a dialogue that transcends time.

➢ **Central Park's Timeless Aura**: Explore how Central Park's lush beauty holds a timeless aura, where yoga becomes a portal to Manhattan's history. It's like stepping into a sanctuary where the city's vibrant pulse meets the serenity of nature.

➢ **Manhattan's Whispers**: Think of yoga as a way to listen to Manhattan's whispered secrets, a language only you and the city understand. Each pose is a moment of deep connection, an unspoken bond with the vivacious soul of Manhattan.

➢ **Yoga Among Skyscraper Silhouettes**: Picture practicing yoga amidst Manhattan's skyscraper silhouettes, where each pose becomes a graceful silhouette against the city's dreams. It's like dancing with the icons that define the skyline.

➤ **Yoga's Harmonious Dialogues**: Explore how yoga becomes a harmonious dialogue, a conversation with the city's many facets. Each pose is a stanza in the poetic exchange between you and Manhattan.

➤ **Sunrise Yoga: Capturing Manhattan's First Light**: Imagine practicing yoga during Manhattan's enchanting sunrise hours, where each pose is a brushstroke on the canvas of the morning sky. It's like becoming part of the city's awakening.

➤ **Yoga as Manhattan's Muse**: Let's talk about how Manhattan itself becomes your muse during yoga practice. It infuses your poses with its energy, its stories, and its relentless pursuit of excellence.

➤ **The Alchemy of Yoga**: Envision yoga as a transformative alchemy, where each pose becomes a potion that blends your essence with Manhattan's. It's a dance of magic and transformation in the heart of the city.

➤ **Reflections in the Glass**: Envision yoga amidst Manhattan's mirrored skyscrapers, where every pose is reflected back—a graceful echo of the city's energy intertwining with your own journey.

➤ **City Pulse Breathing:** Sync each breath with Manhattan's heartbeat, grounding yourself in the city's vibrant rhythm.

In the heart of this magnificent city, where yoga meets the essence of Manhattan, your practice becomes a dance, a meditation, and a profound connection with the city's soul. Embrace it, my darlings, and let your yoga practice become a mesmerizing journey that captures the very essence of Manhattan in The Manhattan Diaries.

Completed Tasks: Metaphysical Yoga Activities

Action Items: Intentions and Thoughts

Yoga As an Anthem

Darlings, welcome to "Yoga as an Anthem." In this dynamic city where every corner holds a story and every moment feels like a verse, we'll explore the art of yoga as an anthem—a melodic connection with Manhattan's vibrant spirit. Picture yourself amidst the iconic landmarks, where yoga becomes a symphony of movement and mindfulness. Join me as we dive into this enchanting chapter, where yoga isn't just about poses; it's about crafting your own anthem that resonates with the heart of Manhattan.

➢ **The Manhattan Symphony**: Imagine, my darlings, that yoga is a symphony, where each pose becomes a note in Manhattan's grand composition. It's like dancing to the vivacious rhythm of the city, with its streets serving as your ballroom.

➢ **Yoga's Dance with Icons**: Picture this: You're practicing yoga amidst Manhattan's iconic landmarks—the dazzling lights of Times Square and the serene beauty of Central Park's Bow Bridge. Your poses become a dance, a waltz, with the city's history and future.

➢ **Yoga's Connection with Manhattan's Essence**: Let's talk about how yoga becomes a profound connection with Manhattan's essence. Each pose is like a stanza in the poetry of the city, an anthem that echoes its ambition, grace, and unwavering spirit.

➢ **Harmonizing with Manhattan**: Think of yoga as a harmonious duet with the ever-changing moods of Manhattan. Each pose is a conversation, a dance that mirrors the city's rich complexity and embraces its highs and lows.

➢ **Flowing Through the City's Rhythm**: Envision each yoga flow as a graceful alignment with Manhattan's rhythm. Your movements echo the city's beat, seamlessly blending strength and serenity in every pose.

➢ **Sunrise Salutations Over the Skyline**: Imagine starting your day with sunrise yoga, as the first light casts a golden glow over the cityscape. Each sun salutation becomes an offering, connecting you with the new day in true Manhattan style.

➢ **Iconic Moments, Inspired Poses**: Think of your yoga practice as an homage to Manhattan's icons—each warrior pose embodies the city's resilience, while tree pose mirrors its unwavering strength amidst the urban landscape.

➢ **Breath of the City**: Picture each inhale as a refreshing embrace of Manhattan's spirit, and each exhale as a release into its vibrant energy. It's a meditation that grounds you within the city's soul.

➢ **Central Park Serenity**: Imagine the calm of practicing yoga in Central Park, the city's green heart. Each pose reflects the balance of urban life and nature's tranquility, making it a true Manhattan anthem in motion.

➢ **Pose with Purpose**: Each yoga pose becomes a tribute to the city's ambition. In every stretch and balance, you're not just moving—you're channeling Manhattan's drive and determination.

➢ **Echoes of the City's Spirit**: With each session, you embody Manhattan's heartbeat. Your practice reflects its dynamism, resilience, and elegance, creating a personal anthem that harmonizes with the city itself.

In the heart of Manhattan, where yoga meets the vibrant cityscape, every pose becomes a dance, a meditation, and a profound connection with the essence of the metropolis. Embrace it, my darlings, and let your yoga practice become a mesmerizing anthem that captures the very soul of Manhattan in The Manhattan Diaries.

Completed Tasks: Yoga Plan Activities

Action Items: Intentions and Thoughts

Finding Your Center in Manhattan

Darlings, welcome to "Finding Your Center in Manhattan." In this bustling city where dreams take shape in the blink of an eye, we'll embark on a journey to discover the art of finding your center through yoga. Picture yourself amidst the iconic Manhattan landmarks, where yoga becomes the compass that guides you through the city's captivating chaos. Join me as we delve into this enchanting chapter, where yoga isn't just about poses; it's about finding your inner sanctuary amidst the vibrant tapestry of Manhattan.

➢ **The Urban Sanctuary**: Imagine, my darlings, that yoga is your urban sanctuary amidst the city's relentless energy. Each pose becomes a moment of serenity, a secret escape from Manhattan's bustling streets, like discovering an oasis in the heart of the metropolis.

➢ **Yoga's Connection with Manhattan's Pulse**: Picture this: You're practicing yoga, and your moves are in perfect sync with Manhattan's pulse—the Vibrant streets, the buzzing energy, and endless possibilities. Your poses become a dance with the city's dynamic heartbeat, an unspoken dialogue with its vivacious spirit.

➢ **Yoga's Resilience**: Let's explore how yoga instills resilience, not just in your body but in your spirit. Each pose is a testament to your inner strength, like the city's enduring resilience in the face of challenges.

➢ **Central Park's Tranquil Embrace**: Think of Central Park as your tranquil embrace amidst the city's chaos. It's where yoga becomes a harmonious dance with nature, like a secret rendezvous with Manhattan's vibrant energy.

➢ **Yoga's Inner Journey**: Envision yoga as an inner journey, where each pose becomes a step towards self-discovery amidst Manhattan's ever-evolving narrative. It's like penning your own story on the canvas of the city.

➢ **Balancing Act**: Picture yoga as the ultimate balancing act, not just in physical postures but in life itself. Each pose becomes a reflection of finding equilibrium amidst the city's dynamic contrasts.

➢ **The Manhattan Mandala**: Let's explore how yoga can create a Manhattan mandala—a vibrant, intricate pattern of movement that mirrors the city's eclectic mix of cultures, dreams, and ambitions.

➢ **Yoga's Empowerment**: Think of yoga as an empowering ritual, where each pose becomes a declaration of your strength and resilience. It's like echoing the city's mantra of "I can" in every breath.

➢ **Meditation in Manhattan**: Imagine practicing yoga as a form of meditation amidst the city's vibrant chaos. Each pose becomes a moment of mindfulness, a way to reconnect with your inner sanctuary.

➢ **Harmony in Hustle:** Visualize each pose as a harmony within the city's relentless hustle. Yoga becomes your way to weave calmness into the whirlwind, grounding you while Manhattan moves around you.

➢ **Power in the Pulse**: Each breath recharges you, drawing strength from Manhattan's energy—a celebration of resilience, echoing the city's unstoppable spirit.

In the heart of Manhattan, where yoga meets the vibrant cityscape, every pose becomes a dance, a meditation, and a profound connection with your inner self. Embrace it, my darlings, and let your yoga practice become a compass that guides you through the captivating maze of The Manhattan Diaries.

Completed Tasks: Finding Your Center Activities

Inspirational Quote

EVEN IF YOU FALL ON YOUR FACE, YOU'RE STILL MOVING FORWARD. — Victor Kiam

Action Items: Intentions and Thoughts

Action Items: Intentions and Thoughts

6

Belvedere Castle Climbs: Staircase Workouts for Royalty in Training

Manhattan, a city that doesn't merely glisten—it gleams, each glint reflecting tales of grandeur, dreams, and an unyielding zeal. Here, amidst a skyline punctuated with spires, it's not only about reaching the top; it's about ascending with allure, elegance, and a touch of royal flair.

Now picture this: You're ascending the steps of Belvedere Castle, every eye irresistibly tracing your climb, not because of the designer of your sneakers, but the undeniable gravity of your grace. That, darling, is the Manhattan Rise to Royalty, an ascent that isn't just about the steps you take, but the majesty with which you take them.

In this captivating chapter of The Manhattan Diaries, we'll explore the art and ardor of the most regal of workouts. From the deliberate, dignified step that channels queens of yore, to the rapid, rhythmic rise of a monarch-in-motion, you'll unearth the secrets of scaling not just staircases, but the summits of your own potential.

But remember, this isn't solely a matter of muscles and might. It's about syncing with the city's spirit, about climbing with a purpose, a legacy, a legend in the making. It's about feeling the weight and wisdom of Manhattan's rich history with each elevation, capturing the essence of its iconic edifices.

Join me, as we feel the pulse of ancient tones and modern metropolis, mastering the climb that not only elevates you but uplifts the very essence of Manhattan with you. Because, sweetheart, in this city, every step upward is a declaration of dominion. Lace up, prepare for your coronation, for the city doesn't just await a performer—it awaits a queen. Welcome to The Manhattan Diaries—where your ascent can mirror the magnificence of Manhattan's most majestic moments.

Climbing in Style: The Manhattan Rise to Royalty

Darlings, let's embark on a royal journey in "Climbing in Style: The Manhattan Rise to Royalty." In the city where dreams ascend as high as the skyscrapers, we'll explore the regal allure of Belvedere Castle Climbs, where each step is a statement of elegance and undeniable grace. Picture yourself as Manhattan's royalty, ascending with majesty against the backdrop of iconic landmarks. Join me as we unveil the secrets of staircase workouts and ascend to new heights amidst the city's splendor.

➢ **The Grand Ascent**: Imagine ascending the steps of Belvedere Castle as a royal procession, with each step exuding regal allure and undeniable grace. It's like stepping into the shoes of Manhattan's royalty, where the city itself becomes your grand palace.

➢ **The Staircase Workout**: Let's dive into the art of staircase workouts, where every step becomes a graceful ascent. From dignified steps that channel queens of old to rapid ascents fit for modern monarchs, it's a workout that combines fitness with finesse.

➢ **A Tribute to Legends**: Journey through the weight and wisdom of Manhattan's rich history with each elevation. Each step carries the essence of the city's iconic edifices, making your climb a tribute to the legends that built Manhattan.

➢ **The Coronation Ascent**: Join me as we prepare for our coronation through the Belvedere Castle climb. In this city, every step upward is a declaration of dominion, and the city itself awaits a queen to mirror its magnificence.

➢ **The Royal Perspective**: Envision the Belvedere Castle climb as your personal royal procession, with each step offering a regal perspective of Manhattan's majestic skyline. It's like ascending the throne of the city.

➤ **Elegance in Every Step**: Explore how every step during the climb exudes elegance and undeniable grace, reminiscent of Manhattan's iconic sophistication.

➤ **Belvedere Castle's Majesty**: Discover the enchanting connection between the climb and Belvedere Castle's majestic allure. Each step becomes a nod to the city's historical splendor.

➤ **A Workout Fit for Queens and Kings**: Delve into the Belvedere Castle climb as a workout that combines the finesse of royalty with the fitness of modernity. It's the ultimate fitness journey in regal style.

➤ **The Grand Coronation**: Join me in preparing for our grand coronation through the ascent. In Manhattan, each step upward is an affirmation of your dominion over your own journey, just as the city itself stands tall in all its magnificence.

➤ **Crowning Moments**: Imagine each pause as a crowning moment, where you soak in Manhattan's panorama as your royal domain. Each view is a reminder that your ascent is not just physical but a rise in spirit and ambition.

➤ **The Final Triumph**: Picture reaching the top as a triumphant coronation. Standing tall, you're not just a climber but Manhattan's royalty, embodying grace and strength against the city's timeless skyline.

In the heart of Manhattan, where each step becomes a royal procession, every ascent is an ode to elegance and undeniable grace. Embrace it, my darlings, for your climb in style is a declaration, an art, and a tribute to the city's enduring grandeur. Welcome to The Manhattan Diaries, where each step mirrors the majesty of Manhattan's most iconic moments.

Completed Tasks: Climbing in Style Activities

Inspirational Quote

NEVER RETREAT. NEVER EXPLAIN. GET IT DONE AND LET THEM HOWL.
— Benjamin Jowett

Action Items: Intentions and Thoughts

Step by Step to Sovereignty: Unveiling the Secrets of Staircase Workouts

Darlings, let's embark on a journey to unveil the secrets of staircase workouts in "Step by Step to Sovereignty." In the city that never sleeps, where dreams ascend as high as skyscrapers, we'll explore the art and ardor of ascending the steps of Belvedere Castle with all the elegance of royalty. Picture yourself as Manhattan's monarch, every step a deliberate and dignified move towards regal fitness. Join me in this workout fit for queens and kings as we unveil the regal side of Manhattan's fitness scene.

➢ **The Regal Ascent**: Envision ascending the steps of Belvedere Castle as a royal procession, each step echoing with the dignity and grace of queens and kings. It's like stepping onto the throne of Manhattan's fitness landscape.

➢ **The Staircase Symphony**: Let's delve into the staircase workout, where each step becomes a note in a regal symphony. From the deliberate steps that channel the grandeur of yore to the rapid, rhythmic rise that suits modern monarchs, it's a fitness routine that combines finesse with strength.

➢ **A Tribute to Manhattan's Legacy**: Explore the weight and wisdom of Manhattan's rich history with each elevation. Every step pays homage to the city's iconic landmarks, turning your workout into a tribute to the legends who built Manhattan.

➢ **The Coronation Climb**: Join me as we prepare for our grand coronation through the Belvedere Castle ascent. In Manhattan, each step upward is a declaration of dominion over your fitness journey, much like the city's declaration of its own majesty.

➤ **The Crown of Confidence**: Discover how the Belvedere Castle climb bestows upon you a crown of confidence. Each step reinforces your regal posture, both in fitness and in life.

➤ **Manhattan's Staircase Legacy**: Immerse yourself in the historical weight of Manhattan's landmarks with each elevation. The climb becomes a tribute to the city's enduring legacy and the architects of its majesty.

➤ **Elevate Your Workout**: Ascend with purpose, for this workout isn't just about building muscles; it's about rising above challenges with grace, much like the city's resilience in the face of adversity.

➤ **Modern Monarchs**: Explore how the rapid, rhythmic rise during the climb captures the essence of modern monarchs. It's a workout that speaks to the strength and agility of today's fitness royalty.

➤ **The Regal Finish Line**: As we conclude our climb, remember that in Manhattan, each step upward is a declaration of dominion. Your coronation isn't just about fitness; it's about embracing the majestic spirit of the city.

➤ **The Throne Awaits**: Picture the top of Belvedere Castle as your throne, where the view is both your reward and your reminder of how far you've come. Each climb is a royal journey, leading to a summit that's as empowering as it is breathtaking.

➤ **Stride of Sovereignty**: Every step echoes Manhattan's strength, claiming your power as you ascend each staircase like a monarch.

In the heart of Manhattan, where each step is a note in a regal symphony, every ascent is an affirmation of your dominion. Embrace it, my darlings, for your climb to sovereignty is a declaration, an art, and a tribute to the city's enduring grandeur. Welcome to The Manhattan Diaries, where each step mirrors the majesty of Manhattan's most iconic moments.

Completed Tasks: Staircase Workouts Activities

Inspirational Quote

IF YOU ARE GOING THROUGH HELL, KEEP GOING. — Winston Churchill

Action Items: Intentions and Thoughts

Manhattan's Staircase Legacy: Climbing Through History

Darlings, let's embark on a captivating journey through Manhattan's Staircase Legacy in this chapter. In the city that breathes history and dreams, we'll explore the art of ascending the steps of Belvedere Castle—an ascent filled with echoes of the city's past and the promise of a majestic future. Picture yourself as a modern monarch, each step an homage to the enduring legacy of Manhattan. Join me in this workout that's not just about fitness but a tribute to the architects of the city's majestic spirit.

➢ **The Regal Ascent**: Imagine the Belvedere Castle climb as your personal royal procession, each step echoing with the dignity and grace of Manhattan's historical figures. It's like stepping into the shoes of a fitness monarch, ascending to your own throne of grandeur.

➢ **Staircase Symphony**: Let's delve into the art of the staircase workout, where every step becomes a note in a symphony of regal fitness. From the deliberate steps reminiscent of bygone eras to the rapid, rhythmic rise fit for modern fitness royalty, it's a workout routine that combines grace with strength.

➢ **Homage to Legends**: Explore the profound connection between your ascent and the rich history of Manhattan. Each step pays homage to the city's iconic landmarks, turning your workout into a tribute to the visionaries who shaped the very essence of Manhattan.

➢ **Climbing with Purpose**: Ascend the stairs with purpose, for this workout isn't merely about building muscles; it's about gracefully rising above challenges, much like the city itself has done throughout its storied history.

➢ **The Grand Coronation**: Join me as we prepare for our grand fitness coronation through the Belvedere Castle climb. In Manhattan, each step upward is a declaration of dominion over your fitness journey, mirroring the city's own declaration of its timeless majesty.

➢ **Elevate Your Confidence**: As you ascend the steps of Belvedere Castle, feel your confidence soar to regal heights. Each step reinforces your posture, both in fitness and in life, transforming you into a more poised and self-assured version of yourself.

➢ **Steps in Time**: Immerse yourself in the history woven into each step of the Belvedere Castle climb. With every ascent, you're not just working out; you're time-traveling through Manhattan's illustrious past, a journey that's as enriching as it is exhilarating.

➢ **A Throne of Fitness**: Picture yourself on a fitness throne, your climb to the top mirroring the ascent of Manhattan's iconic skyline. It's a workout fit for royalty, where you reign as the monarch of your own fitness journey.

➢ **The Monarch's Finish Line**: As we conclude our regal ascent, remember that in Manhattan, each step upward is a proclamation of dominion. Your fitness journey is a testament to your strength, grace, and the majestic spirit of the city itself.

➢ **Crowning Achievement**: As you reach the top, feel the triumph of your journey. This final step isn't just the end of a workout; it's a crowning moment that celebrates Manhattan's resilience and your own regal strength.

In the heart of Manhattan, where every step is a note in a symphony of regal fitness, each ascent is a testament to your dominion. Embrace it, my darlings, for your climb through history is an homage, an art, and a captivating tribute to the enduring legacy of Manhattan. Welcome to The Manhattan Diaries, where climbing through history isn't just a workout—it's a majestic ode to the city's timeless spirit.

Completed Tasks: Climbing Through History Activities

Inspirational Quote

PERSEVERANCE IS FAILING 19 TIMES AND SUCCEEDING THE 20TH. — Julie Andrews

Action Items: Intentions and Thoughts

The Coronation Climb: Becoming Manhattan's Queen

Darlings, in this chapter, we're embarking on a journey of regal proportions—the "Coronation Climb." Picture yourself as Manhattan's reigning queen, ascending the steps of Belvedere Castle with all the elegance and grace of royalty. Every step you take is like a stride toward your fitness throne, where you'll be crowned the queen of your own health and well-being. Join me in this workout that's not just about fitness but about becoming the queen of Manhattan's fitness scene.

- ➤ **The Royal Ascent**: Picture your Belvedere Castle climb as a grand coronation, where each step resonates with the elegance and grace of queens. It's a journey that transcends the mere realm of fitness-it's your path to becoming Manhattan's fitness royalty.

- ➤ **Staircase Elegance**: Delve into the elegance of the staircase workout, where each step becomes a graceful move in your fitness ballet. From deliberate steps that resonate with the past to rhythmic rises that symbolize modern-day queens, it's a workout that marries strength with finesse.

- ➤ **A Tribute to Manhattan**: Ascend with purpose, paying homage to the city's rich history with every step. Just as Manhattan rises above challenges with resilience, your climb embodies the art of gracefully conquering life's obstacles.

- ➤ **The Queen's Coronation**: Join me as we prepare for our fitness coronation through the ascent of Belvedere Castle. In Manhattan, each step upward is more than a personal achievement; it's a tribute to the city's grandeur and enduring spirit.

- ➤ **Elevate Your Confidence**: With every regal step you take, feel your confidence ascend to new heights. Each stride reinforces your posture, both in fitness and in life, transforming you into a more poised and self-assured version of yourself.

➤ **Steps Through Time**: Immerse yourself in the rich history woven into each Belvedere Castle climb. Each step becomes a journey through Manhattan's illustrious past, a workout that's as enlightening as it is exhilarating.

➤ **Claiming Your Throne**: Envision yourself on a fitness throne, ascending with the grace of a queen. Your journey to the top is a regal procession, where you reign as the monarch of your fitness realm.

➤ **The Majesty of Completion**: As we conclude our royal ascent, remember that in Manhattan, every step upward is a proclamation of dominion over your fitness journey. Your climb is a testament to your strength, grace, and the timeless grandeur of the city itself.

➤ **The Queen's Perspective**: As you reach each new height, pause to take in the city's panoramic views—your kingdom stretching out below. It's a reminder that every step brings a fresh perspective, empowering you to rise above with clarity and purpose.

➤ **Crowning Glory**: At the summit, embrace the triumph of reaching your royal peak—your final step a crown of resilience, mirroring Manhattan's enduring spirit.

In the heart of Manhattan, where every step is a journey to dominion, each ascent is a declaration, an art form, and a tribute to the city's lasting legacy. Embrace it, my darlings, for your climb in "The Coronation Climb" is not just a workout-it's your royal path to becoming the queen of your own captivating story. Welcome to The Manhattan Diaries, where grace, elegance, and majesty intertwine with fitness to create a tale as enchanting as Manhattan itself.

Completed Tasks: Coronation Climb Activities

Inspirational Quote

I REALLY BELIEVE THAT EVERYONE HAS A TALENT, ABILITY, OR SKILL THAT HE CAN MINE TO SUPPORT HIMSELF AND TO SUCCEED IN LIFE. — Dean Koontz

Action Items: Intentions and Thoughts

Action Items: Intentions and Thoughts

7

Strawberry Fields Forever
Fit: Toning to the Tunes of Legends

Manhattan, a city that doesn't just hum—it resonates, every chord reverberating tales of icons, aspirations, and unapologetic passion. And in this metropolis of endless beats, it's not only about setting the pace; it's about doing so with rhythm, resonance, and a touch of rock 'n' roll.

Now visualize: You're dancing across Central Park West, every glance irresistibly fixed on you, not due to the chicness of your headphones, but the symphony of your silhouette. That, my dear, is the Manhattan Groove Gala, a dance that's less about steps and more about stories, ones that evoke memories of legends and lyrical lore.

In this electrifying chapter of The Manhattan Diaries, we'll dive deep into the art of moving to Manhattan's most iconic melodies. From the soulful sway reminiscent of timeless ballads to the energetic jumps of pop anthems, you'll learn how to tone while tuning into the city's rich musical heritage.

But let's be clear—it's not just about the calories you burn. It's about harmonizing with the city's soulful soundtrack, moving with a purpose, a playlist, a legacy. It's about balancing the energy of roaring concerts with the serenity of silent sonatas, understanding the highs and lows of Manhattan's melodic heart.

Join me, as we groove to the pulsating rhythms birthed from both underground clubs and grand concert halls, mastering a dance that not only shapes you but shakes the city along with you. Because, darling, in Manhattan, every beat is an invitation to a beautiful ballet. Slide into those dancing shoes; the city is eager for your encore. Welcome to The Manhattan Diaries—where your rhythm can be as resonant as the city's most revered records.

Iconic Moves: Dancing Through Manhattan's Music History

Manhattan, the city where every step becomes a dance move, is a tapestry of iconic melodies that have woven the soundtrack of its history. From the sultry sways of jazz to the rebellious energy of rock 'n' roll, the streets resonate with the rhythms that have defined eras. Join me as we embark on a dance through Manhattan's music history, discovering the iconic moves that have shaped this vibrant metropolis.

➤ **Jazz Syncopation**: Picture yourself in the heart of Harlem, where the sultry rhythms of jazz resonate through dimly lit speakeasies. Here, it's all about the sensuous sway, the syncopation of your hips matching the mesmerizing beat. You become part of the narrative, a dancer in a timeless tale of love and longing.

➤ **Rock 'n' Roll Rebellion**: Feel the electric energy coursing through the Lower East Side's iconic venues, where rock 'n' roll was born. Your moves mirror the wild spirit of rebellion, the music pulsating through your veins as you let loose on the dance floor. It's not just dancing; it's a declaration of independence.

➤ **Broadway Showstopper**: Step into the spotlight of Times Square, where the neon lights illuminate your every move. In the world of Broadway, your dance becomes a story, each step a carefully choreographed moment of magic. You're not just dancing; you're performing a showstopper, captivating the hearts of a captive audience.

➤ **Disco Fever in the Village**: Transport yourself to the glittering dance floors of the Village's legendary disco clubs. As you strut to the funky beats, the disco ball's reflections cascade around you, and you become a vision of the Studio 54 era, where glamour met groove.

➢ **Hip-Hop Hustle**: Embrace the urban pulse of hip-hop on the streets of the Bronx, where this genre was born. Your moves echo the rhythm of the city, each step a testament to the culture and creativity that have defined the borough's identity.

➢ **Latin Heat in Spanish Harlem**: Salsa, merengue, and bachata-immerse yourself in the vibrant Latin rhythms of Spanish Harlem. Your hips sway to the fiery beats, and you become a part of the neighborhood's passionate dance tradition, where every step is a celebration of life and love.

➢ **Indie Rock Revival in Williamsburg**: Cross the bridge to Brooklyn's Williamsburg neighborhood, where indie rock has found its home. Your dance is a fusion of alternative energy and artistic expression, mirroring the neighborhood's eclectic spirit.

➢ **Swingin' Big Band Beat**: Imagine the grand ballrooms of Midtown during the Big Band era, where swing ruled the dance floors. Your feet tap and spin in sync with the brass-heavy tunes, capturing the jubilant spirit of a time when dance and music were a joyful escape.

➢ **Electro Pop Pulse**: Step into the East Village's underground, where electro pop was born. Your moves are sharp and electric, pulsing with Manhattan's nightlife innovation and creativity.

In a city where legends were made and anthems composed, your dance becomes a tribute to its musical heritage. Whether you're swaying to jazz, rocking out to the Lower East Side's beats, or performing a Broadway showstopper, each step resonates with the soul of Manhattan's streets. As you dance through its music history, you become a living chapter in The Manhattan Diaries, where your rhythm is a vibrant ode to the city's iconic tunes. So, lace up those dancing shoes and let's waltz through Manhattan's melodies, where every move is a passionate embrace of its legendary songs.

Completed Tasks: Iconic Music Moves Activities

Action Items: Intentions and Thoughts

Playlist Power: Sculpting Your Body to the Soundtrack of Manhattan

Manhattan, where every street has its own rhythm and every skyline its melody, is a city that dances to the beat of its own drum. But what if I told you that your playlist could become the soundtrack to sculpting not just your moves but your body? Join me as we dive into the magnetic world of Playlist Power, where the songs you choose become the steps to a new you amidst the vibrant cityscape.

➤ **Jazzercise Jams**: Transport yourself to the heart of a jazz club in the Village. With every note, your body sways and twists, sculpting a silhouette as smooth as the saxophone's melody. Jazzercise isn't just a workout; it's an elegant dance through the history of Manhattan's music.

➤ **Rock 'n' Roll Rhythms**: Crank up the volume to the timeless classics of rock 'n' roll. As the electric guitar wails, you move with a wild, untamed spirit, channeling the rebellious energy of Manhattan's rock scene. Your body becomes a canvas of strength and resilience.

➤ **Broadway Beats**: Take center stage in your own fitness musical. Each Broadway showtune carries you through a different scene, from high-energy dance numbers to tender ballads. Your workout transforms into a performance, and every move becomes a moment.

➤ **Hip-Hop Grooves**: Embrace the urban energy of Manhattan's hip-hop scene. Each beat and rhyme fuels your workout, transforming it into a powerful dance of strength and style. Your moves mirror the city's rhythm, and you become a hip-hop hero.

➤ **Latin Dance Fiesta**: Salsa, merengue, and bachata-immerse yourself in the passionate Latin dance vibes of Spanish Harlem. Your body moves to the caliente beats, toning and sculpting as you savor the flavors of Latin music. It's not just a workout; it's a fiesta of fitness.

> **Indie Rock Resilience**: Journey into the indie rock soundscapes of Williamsburg, Brooklyn. With each guitar riff and indie anthem, you find your own rhythm, crafting a workout that's as unique as the neighborhood itself. You're not just sculpting your body; you're shaping your own indie story.

> **EDM Energy Explosion**: Dive into the electronic dance music (EDM) universe of Brooklyn's warehouse raves. The pulsating beats electrify your movements, turning your workout into a high-energy dance party. You're not just sweating; you're raving your way to fitness.

> **Classical Crescendo**: Experience the elegance of Manhattan's classical music heritage. Each symphony and concerto guides your workout with grace and precision. Your body becomes a canvas of classical artistry, as you sculpt with the same finesse as a virtuoso's performance.

> **Pop Anthem Power**: Tune into the catchy beats of pop anthems from Manhattan's biggest stages. Each beat drives you forward, infusing your workout with energy and rhythm. You're not just moving; you're harnessing the upbeat spirit of the city.

In a city where music is life, your playlist becomes a guiding force in your fitness journey. Jazzercise, rock 'n' roll, and Broadway beats all weave together to create the symphony of your transformation. As you sculpt your body to the sounds of Manhattan, you become a living testament to The Manhattan Diaries, where your rhythm is a part of the city's ever-evolving story. So, cue up those tracks and let your playlist power your path to a new you in the heart of Manhattan's iconic streets. Your body, like the city, is a masterpiece in the making.

Completed Tasks: Playlist Power Activities

Inspirational Quote

BE MISERABLE. OR MOTIVATE YOURSELF. WHATEVER HAS TO BE DONE, IT'S ALWAYS YOUR CHOICE. — Wayne Dyer

Action Items: Intentions and Thoughts

The Sound and Silence of Manhattan's Melodies

Manhattan, where every street corner seems to hum with a unique tune, is a city that lives and breathes music. But there's more to the melody than meets the ear. Join me as we venture into the soul of Manhattan's music scene, where the symphony of sounds and the power of silence intertwine to create a mesmerizing story of the city's spirit.

> ➢ **Late-Night Jazz Joints**: Dive into the smoky, dimly lit jazz clubs of the Village. The haunting melodies of saxophones and pianos paint a picture of an era when legends like Miles Davis and Billie Holiday graced these stages. It's not just music; it's a time machine to Manhattan's jazz heyday.

> ➢ **Subway Serenades**: Amidst the hustle and bustle of subway platforms, talented musicians emerge. Their music fills the underground with a diverse array of sounds, from soulful ballads to energetic beats. It's a reminder that in Manhattan, even the everyday commute can become a musical experience.

> ➢ **Silent Central Park**: Amidst the lush greenery of Central Park, there's a unique silence that speaks volumes. The tranquility and stillness allow you to connect with your inner rhythm, whether you're practicing yoga or simply finding solace amidst the city's chaos.

> ➢ **Broadway Brilliance**: Step into the dazzling world of Broadway, where the streets come alive with the magic of musical theater. The energy of Times Square and the grandeur of the theaters make every visit a show-stopping workout in itself.

> ➢ **Harlem's Heritage**: Explore the historical heart of Harlem, where the vibrant sounds of gospel choirs and the rhythm of African drums are a testament to the neighborhood's rich musical legacy. Your

workouts here become a celebration of cultural diversity and the power of music to unite.

➢ **Acoustic Ambiance**: In the cozy cafes of Greenwich Village, acoustic melodies fill the air as emerging artists strum their guitars and share their stories. These intimate settings provide the perfect backdrop for workouts that are as heartfelt as the lyrics being sung.

➢ **The Metropolitan Opera Stairs**: The grand staircase of The Met is not only an architectural wonder but also a place where silence meets splendor. The regal atmosphere inspires workouts that echo the grace and poise of opera stars.

➢ **East River Serenity**: Along the East River, the gentle lapping of water against the shore sets a serene rhythm. It's a place where yoga and meditation are elevated by the calming soundscape of nature, offering a tranquil escape from the city's hustle.

➢ **Rooftop Reverie:** Ascend to one of Manhattan's iconic rooftops, where the city's hum blends with the soft whispers of the wind. Above the bustle, the quiet contrasts with the distant city sounds, creating a serene space where you can reflect, unwind, and embrace the harmony of Manhattan's skyline and spirit.

In a city where every street has a story, jazz joints, subway serenades, and Central Park's serene silence are chapters in the tale of Manhattan's melodies. These sounds and the moments of silence are threads woven into the fabric of The Manhattan Diaries, where your journey is harmonized with the city's timeless soundtrack. Whether you're immersed in the jazz age, inspired by subway buskers, or finding peace in the heart of the park, your connection to Manhattan's music is a testament to the city's enduring allure. As you listen and embrace the silence, you become a part of the city's ever-evolving narrative. Welcome to The Manhattan Diaries-where your personal melody dances to the rhythm of the city's soul.

Completed Tasks: Sound and Silence Activities

Inspirational Quote

BE KIND WHENEVER POSSIBLE. IT IS ALWAYS POSSIBLE. — Dalai Lama

Action Items: Intentions and Thoughts

Dance Your Manhattan Story

Manhattan, a city where dreams are spun into reality, pulsates with the rhythm of countless stories. Amidst its towering skyscrapers and bustling streets, there's a unique narrative waiting to be uncovered — one that's filled with elegance, endurance, and the timeless art of dance. Join me as we step into the world of Manhattan's dance floors and explore how every twirl, dip, and leap becomes a chapter in The Manhattan Diaries.

➢ **Ballet at Bow Bridge**: Embark on a graceful journey reminiscent of a classic ballet. Under the iconic Bow Bridge, your movements mirror the poetry of Manhattan's skyline, creating an exquisite dance of form and function.

➢ **Jazzing Up the Village**: Dive into the heart of Greenwich Village, where jazz and rhythm blend seamlessly. As you dance to the city's vibrant jazz scene, every step becomes a syncopated celebration of the neighborhood's rich history.

➢ **Broadway Brio**: Take center stage in the dazzling world of Broadway. Here, the energy of Times Square infuses your dance with the same enthusiasm that lights up the marquees, making every routine a show-stopping performance.

➢ **Salsa Sensation in Spanish Harlem**: Feel the heat of Spanish Harlem as you immerse yourself in the sensual rhythms of salsa. The vibrant culture and passionate music infuse your dance with a fiery energy that mirrors the neighborhood's essence.

➢ **Contemporary Expressions at The High Line**: On The High Line, Manhattan's elevated park, embrace the freedom of contemporary dance. Against a backdrop of greenery and urban art, your movements become a fusion of creativity and connection with the city's modern soul.

> **Tango at The Battery**: At the southern tip of Manhattan, the Battery Park waterfront offers a perfect setting for the sultry embrace of tango. Dance along the shoreline, where the breeze carries whispers of maritime history, and your tango becomes a passionate tribute to the city's past and present.

> **Hip-Hop Hustle in Harlem**: In the streets of Harlem, where hip-hop was born, channel the rhythm and attitude of this iconic genre. With each step, you pay homage to the neighborhood's contribution to the global music and dance culture.

> **Central Park Swing**: Swing dancing in Central Park is a nostalgic journey back in time. The lush park setting and swinging jazz tunes transport you to the era of the Harlem Renaissance, where swing was king, and your dance tells a story of bygone elegance.

> **Disco Dreams in the East Village**: Step into the East Village, where the vibrant spirit of disco still glitters. Under the neon lights and with echoes of the Studio 54 era, your dance becomes a lively celebration of freedom and flair, capturing the electric pulse of Manhattan's nightlife.

In the dance studios, under the bridges, and amidst the bright lights of Broadway, your journey echoes the city's eclectic spirit. These moments of elegance, jazz-infused energy, and Broadway brio are integral to The Manhattan Diaries, where your story harmonizes with the city's enduring allure. Your dance becomes a part of Manhattan's narrative, capturing the essence of this vibrant metropolis. Whether you're dancing with grace, improvising to jazz, or channeling the brio of Broadway, you're scripting a captivating chapter in The Manhattan Diaries. Welcome to a city where every dance is a chance to author your own story in the heart of Manhattan's grand ballroom.

Completed Tasks: Dance Your Story Activities

Inspirational Quote

THE WILL TO SUCCEED IS IMPORTANT, BUT WHAT'S MORE IMPORTANT IS THE WILL TO PREPARE. — Bobby Knight

Action Items: Intentions and Thoughts

Action Items: Intentions and Thoughts

8

Conservatory Water Cardio: Rowing Your Way to Radiance

Manhattan, a city that doesn't just feel the ripples—it creates the waves, every stroke narrating tales of drive, romance, and undeniable flair. Amidst the sprawling labyrinth of streets, there exists a serene oasis where it's not about pacing on foot but propelling on water—with elegance, vigor, and a touch of the dramatic.

Picture it: You're steering through Central Park's Conservatory Water, every onlooker irresistibly captivated, not by the designer of your attire, but by the grace of your glide. That, darling, is the Manhattan Water Waltz—a dance of oars and reflection that speaks of mastery, allure, and a dash of the unexpected.

In this sparkling chapter of The Manhattan Diaries, we'll set sail into the mystique of Manhattan Rowing. From the seductive pull that mimics a lover's embrace to the dynamic dash of someone chasing dreams, you'll unveil the secrets of navigating life's waters with precision and style.

But let's not be fooled—it's not merely about the arm strength or the rhythm. It's about synchronizing with the city's ebb and flow, about rowing with a mission, a tale, a fervor. It's about the juxtaposition of Central Park's tranquil waters against the city's bustling backdrop, understanding the yin and yang of Manhattan's heartbeat.

Join me, as we embark on this aquatic odyssey, harnessing the energy from both the gentle ripples and roaring currents, perfecting a technique that promises not just fitness, but a splash of enchantment. Because, sweetheart, in Manhattan, every ripple is an opportunity for a mesmerizing ballet on water. Grab your oars, for the city anticipates your next move. Welcome to The Manhattan Diaries—where your row can be as spellbinding as the city's reflections.

The Elegance of Conservatory Water

Amidst Manhattan's bustling energy, there's a tranquil oasis known as Conservatory Water, where elegance and serenity intersect. Here, rowing becomes a dance of grace and precision. Welcome to a chapter of The Manhattan Diaries that unveils the hidden elegance of Conservatory Water in Central Park.

➢ **Central Park's Hidden Gem**: Conservatory Water, nestled within the heart of Central Park, is a hidden gem that beckons those seeking an elegant escape from the city's hustle and bustle. As you glide upon its serene surface, you'll discover that this enchanting waterway is Manhattan's own aquatic oasis.

➢ **Rowing as an Art Form**: Rowing in Conservatory Water isn't just a physical activity; it's an art form. Each stroke of the oar is a brushstroke on the canvas of Manhattan's elegance. The water's stillness reflects the grace of those who choose to row here, creating a mesmerizing spectacle amidst the city's concrete canyons.

➢ **An Escape to Tranquility**: In the midst of Manhattan's relentless energy, Conservatory Water offers a tranquil escape. The surrounding landscape, adorned with blooming flowers and classical statues, transforms your rowing experience into a journey through time and beauty. It's a place where you can momentarily leave the city behind and immerse yourself in the serenity of nature.

➢ **Central Park's Timeless Allure**: Central Park has always been the beating heart of Manhattan's green spaces, a sanctuary where dreams can unfurl. As you row through Conservatory Water, you become part of a timeless narrative, connecting with the park's rich history and the dreamers who have sought solace here for generations.

➤ **Rowing as Poetry**: Picture yourself on the serene Conservatory Water, where rowing becomes a graceful ballet of poetry in motion. Each stroke of the oar tells a story, creating delicate ripples that echo the rhythm of Manhattan's beating heart. In this enchanting setting, rowing transcends mere exercise; it transforms into a captivating performance, where every movement is a stanza in the ballad of elegance.

➤ **The Allure of Central Park**: Dive into the allure of Central Park's Conservatory Water, where the juxtaposition of nature's calm and the city's vibrant energy paints a mesmerizing portrait.

➤ **Elegance Beyond Skyscrapers**: In the heart of Manhattan, elegance takes center stage not only in fashion and architecture but also on the serene waters of Conservatory Water. It's a reminder that beauty can be found in the simplicity of rowing across a tranquil pond, surrounded by lush greenery and the city's timeless charm.

➤ **Finding Zen in Rowing**: Explore how rowing in this tranquil oasis provides a meditative escape from the hustle and bustle of the city, allowing Manhattanites to find their Zen amidst the chaos of their daily lives and discover a sense of Zen through rowing. The rhythmic motion of rowing becomes a meditation, allowing rowers to synchronize with the soothing cadence of nature.

Conservatory Water is more than just a body of water-it's a testament to Manhattan's capacity for elegance and sophistication. As you row upon its gentle ripples, you become a part of the city's ongoing story of grace and beauty. These moments on the water are a chapter in The Manhattan Diaries, where elegance isn't just a concept; it's a way of life. Welcome to The Manhattan Diaries-where your rowing journey becomes a lyrical dance in the heart of Central Park's elegance, mirroring the timeless allure of this iconic Manhattan landmark.

Completed Tasks: Water Activities

Inspirational Quote

IN ORDER TO SUCCEED, WE MUST FIRST BELIEVE THAT WE CAN. — Nikos
Kazantzakis

Action Items: Intentions and Thoughts

Romantic Rowing: A Central Park Love Story

In the heart of Manhattan's bustling urban landscape lies a hidden gem that tells a timeless love story-the enchanting Conservatory Water in Central Park. Picture this: You and your beloved, nestled in a rowboat, gliding across the glistening water, surrounded by the lush greenery of the park. It's a scene straight out of a classic romance novel, where the city's skyscrapers serve as the backdrop to your own love story. In this chapter of The Manhattan Diaries, we dive into the romantic allure of rowing on Conservatory Water, where every stroke of the oar becomes a poetic declaration of love. Let's explore the facets of this love story, from the gentle ripples that mirror your heartbeats to the echoes of laughter that blend with the city's symphony.

➢ **Love on the Water**: There's something undeniably romantic about being on the water, and Conservatory Water offers the perfect setting for couples to escape the urban chaos and embrace the tranquility of nature. Whether it's a first date or a long-standing romance, rowing on this serene pond creates an intimate atmosphere that's perfect for kindling or rekindling love.

➢ **A Scenic Escape**: Amidst the towering skyscrapers of Manhattan, Conservatory Water provides a picturesque escape where you can disconnect from the city's demands and connect with your partner. The view from your rowboat includes the iconic Alice in Wonderland statue, the charming Kerbs Boathouse, and the vibrant tapestry of Central Park-all adding to the romantic ambiance.

➢ **Whispered Secrets**: As you row, you'll find that the gentle lapping of water against your boat seems to encourage whispered confessions and sweet nothings. Conservatory Water becomes a place where couples share their dreams, aspirations, and secrets, creating bonds that deepen with each stroke of the oar.

- ➢ **Central Park Serenade**: While rowing on Conservatory Water, you'll be serenaded by the sounds of Central Park. The laughter of children playing, the rustle of leaves in the wind, and the distant melodies of street musicians create a symphony that accompanies your romantic journey. It's a reminder that even in the heart of the city, moments of serenity and connection can be found.

- ➢ **Timeless Traditions**: Rowing on Conservatory Water is a timeless tradition that has been passed down through generations of Manhattanites. Couples can partake in this age-old practice, connecting with the city's history while forging their own romantic legacy.

- ➢ **The Art of Synchronization**: Rowing requires perfect synchronization between partners, making it a beautiful metaphor for a successful relationship. As you navigate the water together, you'll learn to communicate, cooperate, and move in harmony, strengthening your bond.

- ➢ **Proposal Perfection**: Conservatory Water has witnessed countless proposals over the years, and it's not hard to see why. The serene setting, coupled with the backdrop of Central Park, provides an idyllic stage for popping the question and beginning a new chapter of your love story.

So, whether you're embarking on a romantic adventure or celebrating years of love, Conservatory Water offers a stage for your own Central Park love story. The city's iconic landmarks may define its skyline, but in this tranquil setting, your love story becomes a part of Manhattan's enduring narrative. Embrace the romance, let your love bloom amidst the water lilies, and create memories that will last a lifetime. Welcome to The Manhattan Diaries—where love, like the city itself, knows no bounds.

Completed Tasks: Romantic Rowing Activities

Inspirational Quote

QUALITY IS NOT AN ACT; IT IS A HABIT. — Aristotle

CONSERVATORY WATER CARDIO

Action Items: Intentions and Thoughts

Precision and Style: Mastering Manhattan Rowing Techniques

Manhattan, a city where every stroke creates ripples of elegance and passion. Amidst the towering skyscrapers, there exists a serene oasis where the art of rowing is elevated to an exquisite dance—a blend of precision, style, and a hint of drama. Imagine yourself on Conservatory Water in Central Park, the city's heartbeat reverberating as you glide through its waters. This is the Manhattan Rowing Symphony, where the oars become your conductor's baton, and every movement is a note in a melodious performance.

➢ **The Dance of Oars**: Rowing on Conservatory Water is more than just a workout; it's a dance. Learn how to master the art of propelling your boat with grace and poise, making each stroke a step in a meticulously choreographed routine.

➢ **Central Park Serenity**: Experience the tranquil beauty of Central Park from a unique perspective. Rowing on Conservatory Water allows you to escape the city's hustle and bustle and find solace in the park's serene surroundings.

➢ **A Fitness Elegance**: Rowing is not just about strength; it's about finesse. Discover how this low-impact workout sculpts your body while embracing the elegance of movement, making it a fitness regimen fit for royalty.

➢ **A Tale of Two Waters**: Central Park's Conservatory Water offers a juxtaposition of nature and urban life. Explore how rowing in this iconic location allows you to harmonize with the park's tranquility while being surrounded by the vibrant city.

➢ **Rowing Romance**: Discover how rowing on Conservatory Water has been the backdrop for countless romantic moments. From first dates to proposals, this serene setting adds an extra touch of enchantment to love stories.

- ➢ **Historical Echoes**: Delve into the history of rowing in Central Park, where iconic races and regattas have taken place. Learn about the legacy of rowing in Manhattan and its enduring appeal.

- ➢ **The Zen of Rowing**: Explore the meditative aspects of rowing. Find out how the rhythmic motion and connection with nature can provide a sense of inner peace and mindfulness, making it more than just a physical exercise.

- ➢ **Rowing Gear and Gadgets**: From traditional wooden boats to modern rowing shells, get insights into the equipment and technology used by rowers. Discover the must-have gear and gadgets for rowing enthusiasts.

- ➢ **Rowing Clubs and Communities**: Manhattan boasts a vibrant rowing community. Learn about the rowing clubs and organizations that offer training, events, and camaraderie for both beginners and experienced rowers. Join a community that shares your passion for rowing and the city.

- ➢ **Mastering the Manhattan Glide**: Refine your rowing technique to achieve the "Manhattan Glide"—a seamless, smooth stroke that carries you effortlessly through the water. Each movement becomes a symbol of grace and power, blending the precision of rowing with the city's unmistakable style.

Join me as we embark on a journey through Manhattan's rowing culture, where each stroke is a brushstroke on a canvas, creating a masterpiece of precision, style, and timeless allure. Whether you're seeking a workout, a romantic escape, or a moment of serenity, Conservatory Water offers it all. Row with me, and let's craft a symphony that echoes through the city's heart, leaving a lasting impression on its watery stage. Welcome to The Manhattan Diaries-where your row can be as captivating as a Central Park sunset.

Completed Tasks: Precision and Style Activities

Inspirational Quote

DON'T WATCH THE CLOCK; DO WHAT IT DOES. KEEP GOING. — Sam
Levenson

CONSERVATORY WATER CARDIO

Action Items: Intentions and Thoughts

Navigating Life's Waters: Rowing as Metaphor for Success

Manhattan, a place where dreams and ambitions reach for the sky, resonates with tales of success, determination, and flair. Amidst the towering skyscrapers, there's a serene sanctuary where the art of rowing mirrors life's journey—a rhythmic push forward, a synchronized pull back, and an unwavering drive to reach new horizons. Picture this: You're gliding across Conservatory Water, each stroke not just propelling you through the water but propelling you toward success. That, my dear, is the Manhattan Metaphor in Motion—a dance that embodies the pursuit of excellence, the elegance of endurance, and the allure of achievement.

➢ **Rowing: A Metaphor for Life**: Explore how rowing serves as a metaphor for navigating life's challenges. Discover how the discipline, dedication, and determination required in rowing mirror the qualities needed for success in any endeavor.

➢ **The Synchronized Team**: Rowing isn't just an individual sport; it's a collective effort. Learn about the importance of teamwork, communication, and coordination in rowing and how these skills can be applied to your personal and professional life.

➢ **The Journey of a Thousand Strokes**: Delve into the concept of long-term goals and persistence. Rowing teaches us that success often comes from continuous effort and pushing through setbacks, mirroring the spirit of Manhattan's relentless pursuit of progress.

➢ **Balancing Act**: Rowing requires balance, both physically and mentally. Explore the idea of work-life balance and how finding equilibrium in your pursuits can lead to a more fulfilling and successful life.

➢ **Rowing Lessons from Manhattan**: Manhattan's iconic landmarks, from the Central Park skyline to the historic boathouses, offer lessons that can be applied to rowing and life. Discover the wisdom hidden within the city's landscape.

➤ **Finding Flow in Chaos**: Rowing in the heart of Manhattan teaches us to find a state of flow amidst the bustling city. Discover how this skill can help you navigate life's challenges with grace and poise.

➤ **The Art of Patience**: Rowing requires patience, waiting for the right moment to apply your strength. Explore how patience can be a virtue in both rowing and pursuing your ambitions in the city that demands it.

➤ **Rowing for Wellness**: Learn how rowing is not only a physical workout but also a meditative experience that promotes mental clarity and well-being. Discover the parallels between rowing and the city's pursuit of a balanced lifestyle.

➤ **Central Park Serenity**: Reflect on the tranquility of Central Park and how rowing in this oasis can serve as an escape from the urban hustle. Explore the importance of finding moments of peace in the city's vibrant chaos.

➤ **Rowing Forward**: Each stroke propels you, just as every step in Manhattan opens new doors. Embrace the momentum and seize the city's endless possibilities.

Rowing on Conservatory Water isn't just a sport; it's a metaphorical journey that teaches us about success, teamwork, perseverance, and balance. As we navigate life's waters, let's draw inspiration from the rhythmic strokes and serene setting of Central Park. The Manhattan Metaphor in Motion reminds us that success is a dance, and Manhattan is the perfect partner. Embrace the journey, find your rhythm, and let your rowing experience inspire you to reach new heights in the city that never sleeps.

Completed Tasks: Life's Waters Activities

Inspirational Quote

AIM FOR THE MOON. IF YOU MISS, YOU MAY HIT A STAR. — W. Clement Stone

CONSERVATORY WATER CARDIO

Action Items: Intentions and Thoughts

Action Items: Intentions and Thoughts

Central Park West Weights:
Lifting with the View of Penthouses

9

Manhattan, a city that doesn't just hear the clinks—it feels the force, every rep echoing tales of drive, dedication, and raw determination. In this metropolis of magnificent marvels, it's not just about lifting your spirit—it's about lifting with flair, with purpose, and with a view that most only dream of.

Now, envisage this: You're in Central Park West, the skyline punctuated with penthouses. And as you hoist those weights, every pair of eyes is riveted, not by the brand of your athletic wear, but by the sheer might of your moves. That, my love, is the Manhattan Weighted Waltz—a symphony of strength and skyline, of poise and penthouses.

In this invigorating chapter of The Manhattan Diaries, we'll delve into the world of elite Central Park workouts. From the graceful deadlift that channels a dancer's grace to the power-packed squat of a mogul in making, you'll unravel the finesse of turning fitness into a glamorous affair.

But remember, this isn't merely about the muscles—it's about syncing with Manhattan's rhythm. It's about lifting with a narrative, a legacy, a vision. It's about soaring with both the skyscrapers and the dreams they house, capturing the essence of Manhattan's grandeur and grit.

Join me, as we embrace the pulse of the park, the ambition of its denizens, and perfect an exercise regimen that promises more than just sculpted muscles. For in Manhattan, every lift, every squat, every rep is a testament to one's ambition. Ready your weights, darling, the city is your gym, and every rep is a step closer to your penthouse dream. Welcome to The Manhattan Diaries—where your workout can be as breathtaking as the city's panoramic views.

Sculpting with Style

In the city that never sleeps, where ambition and aspiration thrive, fitness isn't just a routine; it's a statement of style. Welcome to "Sculpting with Style," a chapter in The Manhattan Diaries where we delve into the world of fitness as a fashionable affair. Against the backdrop of iconic Manhattan landmarks, we'll explore how to sculpt your body with grace, confidence, and flair. From chic workout attire to elegant exercise routines, here's how you can make fitness a glamorous part of your Manhattan lifestyle.

- ➢ **Fitness Fashion Finesse**: Elevate your workout attire with Manhattan-inspired style. Discover the perfect blend of function and fashion in activewear that matches the city's vibrancy.

- ➢ **Central Park Serenity**: Find your workout sanctuary amidst the hustle and bustle of Central Park. Unwind and sculpt your body against the tranquil backdrop of the Great Lawn or Jacqueline Kennedy Onassis Reservoir.

- ➢ **Skyline Yoga**: Elevate your yoga practice to new heights as you stretch and meditate against the breathtaking Manhattan skyline. Let the city's energy flow through you as you find your inner zen.

- ➢ **Iconic Sculpture Gardens**: Explore outdoor sculpture gardens like the Storm King Art Center, where fitness and art intersect. Use the sculptures as fitness props and add an artistic flair to your workout routine.

- ➢ **The High Line Hike**: Transform your cardio workout into a scenic adventure by hiking the High Line, an elevated park with lush greenery and stunning views. Get your heart rate up while soaking in the beauty of the city.

➢ **Rooftop Pilates with a View**: Elevate your core strength and flexibility while enjoying panoramic views from one of Manhattan's trendy rooftop Pilates studios. It's fitness with flair, darling.

➢ **Sculpting by the Hudson**: Combine fitness and relaxation with a picturesque riverside jog along the Hudson River Park. The waterfront ambiance adds a touch of tranquility to your workout.

➢ **Stylish Post-Workout Cafes**: Explore Manhattan's chic post-workout cafe scene, where fitness enthusiasts gather to refuel and socialize in fashionable settings. It's where health and style intersect.

➢ **Yoga Retreats in the City**: Discover exclusive yoga retreats held in the heart of Manhattan, where you can escape the urban hustle and find serenity within the city's vibrant energy.

➢ **Nighttime Sculpting**: Step into the enchantment of Manhattan's nighttime workouts, where the city's shimmering lights cast an inspiring glow over your fitness journey. Imagine the skyline as your backdrop, each twinkling light reflecting your determination and drive. Under the moonlit sky, your workout transforms into a rhythmic dance, sculpting not just your body but your spirit amidst the iconic views of Manhattan. It's an experience where strength and elegance meet, and the energy of the city fuels every movement, creating a workout as captivating as the lights around you.

As you sculpt your body in the heart of Manhattan, remember that fitness here isn't just about physical transformation; it's about embracing the city's spirit, making a statement, and leaving your mark on the iconic landscape. Your journey to a more stylish, sculpted self is not just a workout; it's an art form, a love letter to Manhattan itself. So, step out in style, explore the city's fitness hotspots, and let your body become a masterpiece against the backdrop of this captivating metropolis. Welcome to The Manhattan Diaries, where fitness meets fashion, and every workout is a work of art.

Completed Tasks: Sculpting with Style Activities

Inspirational Quote

OPPORTUNITY DOES NOT KNOCK; IT PRESENTS ITSELF WHEN YOU BEAT DOWN THE DOOR. — Kyle Chandler

Action Items: Intentions and Thoughts

CENTRAL PARK'S FITNESS HACKS

Penthouse Motivation

In the glittering world of Manhattan, where aspirations soar higher than skyscrapers, finding your penthouse motivation isn't just a desire—it's a lifestyle. Imagine this: You're in the heart of the city, surrounded by the majestic penthouses of Central Park West. Each weight you lift, every rep you complete, is a step closer to the penthouse dream. It's not just about fitness; it's about sculpting your life with style and purpose amidst the urban splendor. Welcome to a chapter of The Manhattan Diaries that's all about Penthouse Motivation—where fitness meets flair and ambition ascends to new heights.

- ➤ **Central Park West Workouts**: Darling, in this glittering borough, fitness isn't just about the burn; it's about finding your motivation amidst the penthouse dreams of Central Park West. Picture it: the city's elite, surrounded by opulence, sculpting their bodies in style, as if every rep is a brushstroke on the canvas of their dreams.

- ➤ **Glamour in Repetition**: Elevate your fitness game, my dears, by infusing every repetition with the elegance and intent that define Manhattan's penthouse lifestyle. It's not just about pumping iron; it's about sculpting your life with the same precision and grace as the city's high-society dwellers.

- ➤ **Strength with a View**: Imagine the synergy, loves-building your strength while indulging in breathtaking penthouse views. It's a dance of raw power and refined luxury, where your fitness journey meets Manhattan's skyline, and together, they reach for the stars.

- ➤ **Manhattan's High-Life Cafes**: After a rigorous workout, step into Manhattan's high-life fitness cafes, where you can refuel your body and network with likeminded go-getters. It's not just about coffee; it's about brewing success, one conversation at a time.

168

➢ **Penthouse Lifestyle Retreats**: Step into Manhattan's exclusive penthouse fitness retreats, sculpting yourself alongside the city's elite. Each stride takes you closer to the penthouse life you envision, as your fitness journey becomes a testament to ambition in Manhattan's heights.

➢ **Celebrity Personal Trainers**: Rub shoulders with Manhattan's fitness elite and get the star treatment from personal trainers who sculpt the bodies of the borough's finest. It's not just about working out; it's about sweating it out alongside those who train the city's famous physiques.

➢ **Artistic Gym Aesthetics**: Picture this: You're toning up in gyms that double as art galleries, surrounded by Manhattan's creative masterpieces. It's a workout experience that's a fusion of fitness and artistic inspiration, capturing the city's artistic pulse.

➢ **Rooftop Yoga Retreats**: Elevate your yoga practice, quite literally, with rooftop sessions that offer sweeping views of the city. It's about finding serenity amidst the urban hustle and bustle, as you flow through your asanas high above the city streets.

➢ **Fitness Concierge Services**: Imagine a fitness concierge tailoring your workouts, nutrition, and wellness to perfection—a personal guru guiding you to penthouse-level fitness with the ease of an Upper East Side stroll.

In Manhattan, fitness is not just about building muscles; it's about forging a path to success that leads straight to the penthouse of your dreams. Your every lift, squat, and rep resonates with the rhythm of the city, reminding you that in this urban jungle, every step toward your goals is a stride toward a life of luxury. So, darling, keep sculpting, keep striving, and let your fitness journey be a testament to your ambition amidst the penthouse-rich landscape of Manhattan.

Completed Tasks: High Rise Motivation Activities

Action Items: Intentions and Thoughts

The Power of Elevation

Manhattan, a city that doesn't just reach for the stars—it creates them, with each ambition, each ascent, and every heart-pounding elevation. In this concrete jungle where dreams are woven into the very fabric of the skyline, it's not just about the journey; it's about rising with sophistication, style, and the thrill of elevation. Picture this: You're scaling heights that touch the clouds, and every onlooker is drawn to you, not by the brand of your sneakers, but the majesty of your ascent. That, my love, is the Manhattan Power of Elevation—a symphony of strength and skyline, of grace and grandeur.

> ➤ **Rooftop Retreats**: Immerse yourself in the rarefied air of Manhattan's rooftop fitness sanctuaries, where the city's skyline becomes your personal canvas. It's not just about breaking a sweat; it's about rising above the ordinary, savoring the views, and sculpting your body amidst this urban oasis in the clouds.

> ➤ **High-Altitude Spinning**: Feel the pulse of the city beneath your feet as you embark on a spinning journey that touches the sky. It's not just about pedaling; it's about the exhilaration of reaching new heights, the city's energy pushing you to go further, faster, and higher.

> ➤ **Sky-High Yoga Sessions**: Elevate your yoga practice both physically and spiritually in the penthouse suites that offer a serene escape from the city's hustle. It's about finding inner peace while being cradled in the arms of Manhattan's dazzling skyscrapers, a true union of the soul and the city.

> ➤ **Elevator Fitness Trainers**: Train like Manhattan's elite with fitness experts who understand that it's not just about lifting weights but elevating your entire fitness journey. They sculpt your body while

helping you reach new heights in sophistication and strength, mirroring the city's grandeur.

➢ **Summit Sunset Runs**: Wrap up your day with an evening run along Manhattan's highest peaks, where the city's skyline transforms into a mesmerizing tapestry of lights. Each stride becomes a statement of ambition, and the skyline is not just a backdrop but your stage. Welcome to The Manhattan Power of Elevation, where you embrace the city's elegance, define your own style, and become the star of your own story, with the skyline as your canvas.

➢ **Penthouse Pilates Precision**: Discover the art of Pilates in exclusive penthouse studios, where precision and poise meet panoramic views. It's not just about core strength; it's about aligning your body and spirit with the grace of the city's architecture, finding balance amidst the bustling metropolis.

➢ **Rooftop Meditation Retreats**: Elevate your mindfulness practice to new heights with guided meditation sessions on the city's rooftops. It's about finding serenity amidst the urban chaos, allowing Manhattan's rhythm to become your mantra, and achieving a sense of calm that transcends the ordinary.

In the heart of Manhattan, where ambition soars as high as the skyline, The Manhattan Power of Elevation is more than a workout—it's an experience. Each rooftop, each summit, every sunlit stretch and moonlit moment becomes a reflection of your journey to rise above the ordinary. With every spin, stride, and stretch, you're not just moving; you're making Manhattan your own, crafting a narrative that melds strength with sophistication and grace with grandeur. Embrace the city's rhythm as your own, and let each elevation become a testament to your ambition, style, and the boundless potential of your story amidst Manhattan's iconic skyline. Welcome to a journey where every ascent leaves a legacy.

Completed Tasks: Elevation Activities

Inspirational Quote

YOU SIMPLY HAVE TO PUT ONE FOOT IN FRONT OF THE OTHER AND KEEP GOING. PUT BLINDERS ON AND PLOW RIGHT AHEAD. — George Lucas

Action Items: Intentions and Thoughts

Central Park's Open-Air Gym

In the heart of Manhattan, where the city's relentless energy meets the tranquility of nature, lies a hidden gem that encapsulates the essence of fitness, finesse, and the allure of Central Park. Welcome to "Central Park's Open-Air Gym," where the lush greenery becomes your backdrop, and your workouts become a harmonious dance with the city's spirit. In this captivating chapter of The Manhattan Diaries, we'll explore the unique charm of exercising amidst the park's natural beauty, where every breath is a testament to your vitality, and every movement is a celebration of Manhattan's grandeur.

- ➢ **Lakeside Yoga Retreat**: Find your inner peace and strength with lakeside yoga sessions that embrace the serenity of Central Park's waters. It's not just about the poses; it's about syncing your breath with the gentle ripples, feeling the earth beneath your mat, and immersing yourself in a holistic experience that transcends the bustling city.

- ➢ **Trail Running Adventures**: Embark on invigorating trail runs through winding paths that offer both a physical challenge and a scenic escape. It's not just about the mileage; it's about discovering hidden corners of Central Park, where the beauty of nature complements the vigor of your stride.

- ➢ **Riverside Cycling Expeditions**: Hop on a bike and explore the park's picturesque riverside trails, where the city's skyline frames your journey. It's not just about cycling; it's about embracing the freedom of the open road, feeling the wind in your hair, and experiencing Manhattan from a unique vantage point.

- ➢ **Picnic Pilates Parties**: Combine fitness and leisure with picnics that include rejuvenating Pilates sessions amidst Central Park's lush lawns. It's not just about the exercises; it's about nourishing your body and soul, enjoying gourmet treats, and sharing moments of wellness with friends against the backdrop of iconic Manhattan landmarks.

➤ **Sculpting with a View**: Elevate your strength training routine with outdoor workouts that make the city's skyline your gym. It's not just about lifting weights; it's about sculpting your body while gazing at the majestic skyscrapers, letting the urban ambiance infuse your determination.

➤ **Tai Chi Tranquility**: Discover inner balance and serenity with Tai Chi sessions set against the backdrop of Central Park's natural beauty. It's not just about the movements; it's about connecting with the park's timeless energy and finding harmony amidst the city's hustle and bustle.

➤ **Sunrise Meditation Retreats**: Start your day with guided meditation sessions that immerse you in the peaceful ambiance of Central Park at sunrise. It's not just about relaxation; it's about finding clarity and purpose as you meditate amidst the awakening city.

"Central Park's Open-Air Gym" invites you to embrace the harmony of fitness and nature, where every workout becomes a symphony of vitality. As you stretch, run, cycle, and sculpt amidst the park's beauty, you're not just enhancing your physical well-being; you're also becoming a part of Manhattan's timeless story. Your journey is a testament to your commitment to health and your appreciation for the city's enduring allure, where Central Park's vibrant energy and Manhattan's landmarks intertwine seamlessly. Welcome to The Manhattan Diaries—where your fitness journey mirrors the grandeur of the city itself, and every session is a step towards a healthier, more vibrant you.

Completed Tasks: Open-Air Workout Activities

_____

_____

_____

_____

_____

_____

_____

_____

_____

_____

_____

_____

_____

_____

_____

_____

_____

_____

_____

_____

_____

_____

_____

_____

_____

_____

_____

Inspirational Quote

IF YOU WANT TO SUCCEED, YOU SHOULD STRIKE OUT ON NEW PATHS, RATHER THAN TRAVEL THE WORN PATHS OF ACCEPTED SUCCESS. — John D. Rockefeller

Action Items: Intentions and Thoughts

CENTRAL PARK'S FITNESS HACKS

Strength and the City

Manhattan, a city that never sleeps, thrives on power-power lunches, power deals, and, of course, the power of strength. Amidst the towering skyscrapers and bustling streets, there exists a realm where strength isn't just about lifting weights; it's about forging a connection with the city's relentless spirit. Imagine this: You're in Central Park, surrounded by the iconic skyline, sculpting your body with every determined rep. That, my dear, is the Manhattan Muscle Melody—an ode to endurance, elegance, and an unyielding drive.

➢ **Skyline Sculpting**: Elevate your fitness routine with outdoor workouts that transform Manhattan's skyline into your backdrop. It's not just about lifting weights; it's about feeling the city's pulse and pushing your limits against its magnificent silhouette.

➢ **Central Park Yoga Retreats**: Find tranquility amidst the urban chaos with yoga sessions held in Central Park's serene corners. It's not just about poses; it's about syncing your breath with the city's rhythm and discovering inner strength through the practice.

➢ **Rooftop Pilates**: Take your core-strengthening exercises to new heights—literally. Rooftop Pilates sessions offer a unique perspective of the city while enhancing your flexibility and balance. It's not just about toning your body; it's about reaching new heights in your fitness journey.

➢ **Cycling Through History**: Explore Manhattan's historic landmarks on a cycling adventure that combines cardio with sightseeing. It's not just about pedaling; it's about immersing yourself in the city's rich narrative while staying active.

➢ **Manhattan Marathon Training**: Join a community of runners as you prepare for the ultimate challenge —the Manhattan Marathon.

It's not just about distance; it's about the endurance, camaraderie, and the thrill of crossing the city's iconic finish line.

➢ **High-Intensity Interval Training (HIIT) on the High Line**: Experience a heart-pounding workout on the elevated High Line park, where HIIT sessions combine urban scenery with intense bursts of exercise. It's not just about sweating it out; it's about pushing your limits while overlooking Manhattan's urban beauty.

➢ **Tai Chi by the Waterfront**: Practice the ancient art of Tai Chi by the Hudson River, finding balance and serenity amidst the city's hustle. It's not just about graceful movements; it's about aligning your energy with the flowing currents of the river and Manhattan's dynamic pace.

➢ **Dance Fusion Classes at DUMBO**: Unleash your inner dancer in DUMBO's open spaces with fusion dance classes that blend various styles. It's not just about choreography; it's about expressing yourself through movement against the backdrop of Brooklyn Bridge and Manhattan's skyline.

➢ **Brooklyn Bridge Boot Camp**: Challenge your body with a boot camp workout on the iconic Brooklyn Bridge. It's not just about drills; it's about conquering while sculpting your physique.

Strength and the City beckon you to redefine fitness amidst the dynamic energy of Manhattan. As you sculpt, stretch, cycle, and run against the city's mesmerizing backdrop, you're not just building physical resilience; you're becoming a part of Manhattan's enduring story. Your journey mirrors the tenacity of the city itself, where Central Park's tranquility and Manhattan's landmarks blend seamlessly. Welcome to The Manhattan Diaries—where your fitness odyssey is a testament to the city's unwavering spirit, and every stride, every pose, every lift, is a step towards a stronger, more empowered you in the heart of this magnificent metropolis.

Completed Tasks: Strength and the City Activities

Inspirational Quote

PERSEVERANCE IS NOT A LONG RACE; IT IS MANY SHORT RACES ONE AFTER THE OTHER. — Walter Elliot

Action Items: Intentions and Thoughts

Action Items: Intentions and Thoughts

The Ramble Routines:
Fitness Trails Amidst Nature's Finest

Manhattan, a city that doesn't just perceive the rustle—it feels the rhythm, as each jog, each sprint echoes tales of zeal, passion, and unbridled spirit. In this steel-and-stone jungle, it's not only about escaping the cacophony—it's about finding serenity, even in the heart of the hustle, with elegance, flair, and a zest for life.

Now, picture this: You're darting through The Ramble, Central Park's enchanting woodland, with every eye discreetly watching, not because of the brand of your sneakers, but by the mesmerizing sync of your steps with nature's heartbeat. That, darling, is the Manhattan Nature Navigating—a dance of dynamism that marries city sophistication with woodland wonder.

In this lush chapter of The Manhattan Diaries, we'll explore the sanctuaries amidst skyscrapers. From the gentle jog that synchronizes with the whispering leaves to the sprint that races with the fleeting deer, you'll learn the art of merging fitness with nature's finesse.

But don't be mistaken—this isn't just about a sprint or jog. It's about entwining with the city's green soul, about running with a purpose, an aura, a fervor. It's about harmonizing with both the wilderness and the wonders they nestle within, grasping the yin and yang of Manhattan's vibrant veins.

Join me, as we trace the paths less traveled, the trails that teem with tales, and master the art of a run that doesn't just exhilarate you, but ensnares the very spirit of Manhattan. For in this city, every pace, every breath, every heartbeat, is a silent symphony waiting to be explored. Lace up those shoes, darling, because Central Park's Ramble beckons. Welcome to The Manhattan Diaries—where your run can be as mesmerizing as the city's secret sanctuaries.

Central Park's Ramble Retreat

Amidst Manhattan's ceaseless rhythm, a hidden gem awaits, offering a sanctuary of serenity and fitness: Central Park's Ramble. Picture this: Your sneakers lightly caress woodland trails, drawing the eyes of onlookers not to logos but to the mesmerizing dance between your footsteps and nature's heartbeat. This is the Manhattan Nature Navigating, where urban sophistication waltzes gracefully with woodland wonder. In this lush chapter of The Manhattan Diaries, let's delve into the secrets of this captivating retreat, where fitness meets nature's finesse, turning every jog into a symphony.

➢ **Exploring the Woodland Trails**: Wander through the enchanting paths of Central Park's Ramble, where you can escape the urban hustle and embrace the tranquility of nature. Lose yourself in the lush greenery, and let the winding trails lead you on a journey of discovery.

➢ **Wild Encounters**: As you jog through this hidden oasis, be prepared for delightful surprises. From playful squirrels darting among the trees to the graceful deer that occasionally cross your path, you'll share your run with the park's diverse wildlife, creating a unique and exhilarating experience.

➢ **Fitness Fusion**: Central Park's Ramble isn't just a place for a workout; it's where you'll learn the art of melding running with nature's finesse. Enhance not only your physical fitness but also your mental well-being as you find harmony with the natural world.

➢ **Green Oasis**: In the heart of the city that never sleeps, discover an oasis of greenery. Immerse yourself in the lush surroundings, breathing in the fresh air and experiencing a sense of calm that can only be found in this hidden corner of Central Park.

THE RAMBLE ROUTINES

> **A Symphony of Strides**: As your feet rhythmically pound the trails, you'll discover that each stride is a note in the symphony of Manhattan. Your run captures the essence of the city, where every step harmonizes with its vibrant rhythm, making your fitness journey a captivating tale of elegance and allure.

> **Meditative Moments**: Amidst the Ramble's tranquility, discover moments of meditation and self-reflection. The winding trails and rustling leaves create the perfect backdrop for finding inner peace and clarity while you run.

> **Seasonal Splendor**: Experience the changing seasons in all their glory as you navigate Central Park's Ramble. From the vibrant colors of autumn to the fresh blooms of spring, each visit offers a different visual feast that enhances your run.

> **Inspiring Artistry**: Along the trails, you'll encounter sculptures and art installations that add a touch of creativity to your run. Let these artistic expressions inspire you as you weave your way through this living masterpiece.

> **Hidden Treasures**: Explore the hidden nooks and crannies of the Ramble, where surprises and discoveries await. Whether it's stumbling upon a secluded bench with a breathtaking view or finding a hidden pond, each run is an adventure filled with unexpected delights.

As you lace up your shoes and embark on this enchanting journey, remember that in Manhattan, every pace, breath, and heartbeat is a silent symphony waiting to be explored. Central Park's Ramble beckons, offering an opportunity to make your run as mesmerizing as the city's secret sanctuaries. Welcome to The Manhattan Diaries, where your fitness journey is a tale of elegance and allure, intertwined with the pulse of the metropolis.

Completed Tasks: Ramble Retreats Activities

Action Items: Intentions and Thoughts

Meditative Running

In the city that never sleeps, the relentless pace can leave you yearning for moments of serenity and introspection. But what if I told you that amidst the hustle and bustle of Manhattan, there exists a unique way to find inner peace, to reconnect with yourself, and to discover the beauty of the urban landscape in a whole new light? Welcome to the world of "Meditative Running," a practice that infuses the energy of the city with the tranquility of meditation, all while you explore iconic Manhattan landmarks.

- ➤ **Riverside Reverie**: Begin your meditative journey along the Hudson River Greenway. As you run alongside the glistening waters with the Statue of Liberty in the distance, let the rhythmic sounds of the waves soothe your soul.

- ➤ **Central Park Serenity**: Head into Central Park, where the Ramble offers a secluded oasis amidst the city's chaos. The winding paths, hidden waterfalls, and vibrant foliage create a meditative haven right in the heart of Manhattan.

- ➤ **Brooklyn Bridge Bliss**: Cross the iconic Brooklyn Bridge, feeling the bridge's history beneath your feet and absorbing breathtaking views of the skyline. The bridge's gentle sway becomes a moving meditation, aligning you with the city's flow.

- ➤ **High Line Harmony**: Explore the High Line, an elevated park that combines lush greenery with contemporary art. Your run becomes a dance through nature and culture, offering a unique blend of tranquility and stimulation.

- ➤ **Financial District Reflection**: Wind down your run in the Financial District. As you pass the Charging Bull and reflect on the city's financial prowess, you'll find a sense of grounding and purpose amidst the urban jungle.

➤ **Empire State of Mind**: Ascend the Empire State Building before sunrise for a meditative run like no other. As the sun emerges on the horizon, casting its golden glow across the city, you'll feel a profound connection with the world below. This breathtaking moment is a reminder that amidst the city's towering skyscrapers, there's a serene beauty that can elevate your spirit.

➤ **Metropolitan Museum Musings**: Explore the steps of The Met, where art and culture converge. Running up and down the grand staircase, surrounded by artistic masterpieces, creates a meditative rhythm that resonates with the city's creative heartbeat. It's a blend of physical exertion and artistic inspiration.

➤ **East River Enlightenment**: Along the East River Esplanade, find a quiet stretch where you can pause and meditate. As the river flows beside you and the city skyline stretches out in both directions, take a moment to reflect on the constant movement and evolution of life in Manhattan.

➤ **Times Square Tranquility**: Believe it or not, Times Square can offer a unique form of meditative running. Amidst the neon lights and bustling crowds, find your own rhythm. As you navigate the lively streets, you'll discover that even in the midst of chaos, you can find moments of stillness within yourself.

Meditative Running in Manhattan is more than just a workout; it's a spiritual journey through the city's diverse landscapes. It's about finding moments of calm amidst the chaos, and with every step, discovering that the city itself can be your most profound meditation guide. So lace up your running shoes, breathe in the city's energy, and embark on a meditative journey that will not only transform your fitness but also your relationship with Manhattan's vibrant soul. Welcome to The Manhattan Diaries, where your run is a path to inner peace amidst the city's symphony of life.

Completed Tasks: Meditative Running Activities

Inspirational Quote

I ATTRIBUTE MY SUCCESS TO THIS—I NEVER GAVE OR TOOK ANY EXCUSE.
— Florence Nightingale

Action Items: Intentions and Thoughts

CENTRAL PARK'S FITNESS HACKS

Wildlife Workouts

Manhattan, a concrete jungle that pulses with life, is home to a different kind of fitness experience-one that brings you closer to nature amidst the city's hustle and bustle. In this chapter of The Manhattan Diaries, we'll venture into the world of "Wildlife Workouts." These fitness routines are unlike any other, allowing you to connect with the wild and awaken your primal instincts, all while surrounded by the iconic landmarks that define Manhattan's skyline.

➤ **Central Park Safari**: Embark on a run through Central Park, where you'll encounter a surprising variety of wildlife. From squirrels scurrying through the trees to vibrant birdlife gracing the park's ponds, every step is a reminder that even in the heart of the city, nature's beauty thrives.

➤ **Riverside Serenity**: Along the Hudson River Greenway, you'll find an oasis where the river meets the city. Take a moment to appreciate the graceful dance of seagulls and the serene presence of swans. It's a wildlife-inspired workout that harmonizes with the tranquil waters.

➤ **Inwood's Avian Adventure**: Explore Inwood Hill Park, the city's last natural forest. Here, you'll encounter an array of bird species, including red-tailed hawks and woodpeckers. Running through this verdant haven will awaken your senses and remind you of Manhattan's wild side.

➤ **East River Encounters**: Along the East River Esplanade, keep an eye out for cormorants and egrets, which gracefully navigate the river's currents. Your workout becomes a peaceful rendezvous with these aquatic wonders, all while surrounded by the city's energy.

➤ **Harlem River Wildlife**: Explore the Harlem River waterfront, where you can spot turtles sunning themselves on rocks and various waterfowl like ducks and geese. Running here offers a peaceful retreat from the city's commotion, surrounded by the soothing sounds of the river and its inhabitants.

➤ **Morningside Heights Birds**: Morningside Park is a birdwatcher's delight, with sparrows, robins, and cardinals filling the air with their songs. Your jog through this park will be a harmonious blend of cardio and avian melodies, a perfect fusion of nature and fitness.

➤ **Tompkins Square Critters**: Tompkins Square Park in the East Village is a haven for dog owners, and your workout may include playful encounters with furry friends and their owners. The cheerful atmosphere and joyful barks will infuse your run with boundless energy.

➤ **Bryant Park Squirrels**: While enjoying a jog around Bryant Park, don't forget to admire the park's agile squirrel population. Their acrobatics in search of food will inspire you to add agility and balance exercises to your workout routine.

➤ **Battery Park's Coastal Touch**: Workout by the waterfront with breezes and glimpses of fish, crabs, and seabirds, bringing a refreshing coastal vibe to your routine.

Wildlife Workouts in Manhattan are a testament to the city's incredible diversity. Amidst the towering skyscrapers and bustling streets, you can find solace and wonder in the presence of wildlife. These unique fitness experiences will not only invigorate your body but also reconnect you with the natural world. Manhattan, with its juxtaposition of urban vibrancy and natural beauty, invites you to embrace the wild and incorporate it into your fitness routine. So, let the city's wildlife be your workout companions and rediscover the enchantment of Manhattan through their eyes. Welcome to The Manhattan Diaries, where every run is an encounter with the untamed soul of the city.

Completed Tasks: Wildlife Workouts Activities

Inspirational Quote

LIFE IS LIKE A TRUMPET—IF YOU DON'T PUT ANYTHING INTO IT, YOU DON'T GET ANYTHING OUT OF IT. — William Christopher Handy

Action Items: Intentions and Thoughts

The Ramble Rhythms

In the heart of bustling Manhattan lies a hidden gem, a place where the city's relentless rhythms seamlessly merge with the tranquil cadence of nature. Central Park's Ramble is a sanctuary for those seeking respite from the urban hustle while indulging in the therapeutic embrace of Mother Nature. Imagine embarking on a jog where every step carries you deeper into a world where towering skyscrapers give way to the lush canopy of trees, and the city's cacophony fades into the melodious chirping of birds. Welcome to The Manhattan Diaries' exploration of "The Ramble Rhythms," where we invite you to lose yourself in the wild beauty of Manhattan's cherished oasis.

> ➤ **Woodland Whispers**: As you tread along the winding paths of the Ramble, the gentle rustle of leaves and the symphony of birds will serenade your senses. It's not just a run; it's a dance with nature, where every stride takes you closer to the park's hidden treasures.

> ➤ **The Birdwatcher's Ballet**: The Ramble is a paradise for birdwatchers. With over 230 species of birds, your jog becomes a ballet of observation. Keep an eye out for the vibrant plumage of warblers and the majestic flight of red-tailed hawks soaring above the city's skyline.

> ➤ **Untamed Serenity**: Amidst the Ramble's dense foliage, you'll encounter serene glens and meandering streams. Pause for a moment of meditation or simply revel in the untouched beauty of these hidden pockets of tranquility.

> ➤ **Art in the Wild**: Nature meets art as you stumble upon the sculptures and ornate bridges that dot the Ramble. These unexpected encounters infuse your run with a touch of culture, reminding you that even in the wild heart of Manhattan, art finds its place.

➢ **The Ramble's Resilience**: Learn from the Ramble's resilience as it bounces back from the challenges of time and weather. Just like the Ramble, you too can overcome obstacles, adapt to change, and emerge stronger with every run.

➢ **Seasonal Sonata**: The Ramble transforms with the seasons, offering a new experience with each visit. From vibrant autumn foliage to the tranquility of a snow-blanketed landscape, your runs become a reflection of nature's ever-changing artistry.

➢ **Flora and Fauna Encounter**: Keep an eye out for the Ramble's diverse flora, from native plants to exotic blooms. As you jog, you might cross paths with curious squirrels, playful chipmunks, or even the occasional deer, reminding you that even in the heart of the city, a touch of the wild awaits.

➢ **Historical Echoes**: The Ramble holds historical significance, and along your route, you'll encounter remnants of a bygone era. Stumble upon the rustic arches, bridges, and structures that harken back to the park's early days and discover the tales they whisper.

➢ **A Photographer's Paradise**: Whether you're a seasoned photographer or just have a smartphone, the Ramble's picturesque landscapes provide countless opportunities to capture the magic of the moment.

The Ramble Rhythms offer more than just a fitness journey; they invite you to harmonize with the untamed soul of Manhattan. With each run through this enchanting woodland, you'll uncover the city's wild side, where skyscrapers and sparrows coexist, and where the urban jungle converges with nature's sanctuary. So, slip on your running shoes, let the Ramble's rhythms guide your stride, and embark on an adventure where Manhattan's heart beats in sync with the wild. Welcome to The Manhattan Diaries, where every jog is a journey of discovery.

Completed Tasks: Strength Training Activities

Inspirational Quote

DOING WHAT YOU LOVE IS THE CORNERSTONE OF HAVING ABUNDANCE IN YOUR LIFE. — Wayne Dyer

Action Items: Intentions and Thoughts

Action Items: Intentions and Thoughts

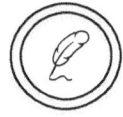

City Roundup: Manhattan Mystiques – From Dreams to Discipline

As we conclude this exhilarating journey through the vibrant tapestry of Manhattan's fitness secrets in "Central Park's Fitness Hacks: How NYC's Best Shape Up," we find ourselves at the intersection of aspiration and achievement, much like this city itself. Each chapter has been a revelation, a glimpse into the lives of those who have mastered the art of sculpting not just their bodies but their destinies.

From the pulse-pounding workouts along Central Park's Jacqueline Kennedy Onassis Reservoir to the graceful ballet sessions by the iconic Bow Bridge, we've witnessed the fusion of strength and grace, much like Manhattan's ever-evolving skyline. The yoga sessions amidst the skyscrapers and the soothing rowing routines on Conservatory Water have taught us that amidst the urban chaos, serenity can always be found.

Our exploration of Central Park's hidden gems, from the secluded Ramble to the open-air gym at Sheep Meadow, has been an ode to the city's innate ability to offer solace and tranquility to those who seek it. And the final revelation, the penthouse workouts overlooking Central Park West, reminded us that in Manhattan, dreams reach heights that are as boundless as the sky itself.

In this city, where ambition knows no bounds, each fitness regimen has been a metaphor for the relentless pursuit of excellence. These workouts aren't just about physical transformation; they're about embracing the essence of Manhattan, with its dreams, aspirations, and relentless drive. We've seen that in every movement, every rep, and every breath, Manhattan's spirit thrives.

So, dear readers, as we conclude our journey through the pages of "Central Park's Fitness Hacks," I urge you to take these lessons to heart. Unravel your inner self, just as we've unraveled the mysteries of Manhattan.

Embrace the energy, the diversity, and the boundless potential that this city offers. Let your own story become a part of the Manhattan mystique, where the skyline is not just a view but a reminder that the possibilities are limitless. Welcome to The Manhattan Diaries, where your journey is just beginning, and the city is your ultimate muse.

Central Park's Fitness Hacks Recap Checklist

The Manhattan Diaries program series recap checklist—completes step seven of your 21 step journey. Think of this program as a time release supplement that does its magic over the course of 21 steps, days, or weeks— you set your schedule. By committing to one chapter each morning—or one book each day or week; in 21 short days or weeks you will be able to change your life into a new You. In this book, we covered:

1. The Bethesda Bootcamp: Sculpting Dreams by the Terrace

In "The Bethesda Bootcamp: Sculpting Dreams by the Terrace," we delve into the transformative power of fitness against the iconic backdrop of Central Park's Bethesda Terrace. Here, each sprint and stretch is more than a workout; it's a commitment to becoming the best version of oneself. This chapter explores the Bethesda Burn, where the city's energy fuels not only physical strength but also inner resolve. With rituals that range from heart-pounding hill sprints to serene cool-downs, this bootcamp represents a journey of self-sculpting—a dedication to dreams, ambition, and resilience that resonates with the spirit of Manhattan.

2. Green Lawn Lunges: Toning Thighs with Every Sunset View

In "Green Lawn Lunges: Toning Thighs with Every Sunset View," we explore the elegance of fitness as an art form, set amidst the lush expanses of Central Park. This chapter transforms lunges into a graceful dance against Manhattan's skyline, each movement merging strength and poise as you embrace the city's unique rhythm. It's not just about the physical benefits; it's a celebration of purpose and passion, capturing balance and beauty under the setting sun. With each lunge, you're not only sculpting your body but weaving yourself into Manhattan's timeless narrative, embodying the sophistication of the city itself.

3. Reservoir Runs: Jogging Tips from Manhattan's Marathoners

In "Reservoir Runs: Jogging Tips from Manhattan's Marathoners," this chapter explores the art of running along Central Park's Reservoir, where Manhattan's elite marathoners share their secrets for turning every jog into an inspiring journey. Beyond the technique, it's about capturing the city's pulse—syncing each stride with the rhythm of New York's ambition and resilience. Here, running is more than exercise; it's a moving ode to Manhattan's dreams and tenacity, where every step tells a story. Lace up and let the city's energy propel you forward, for in The Manhattan Diaries, every run becomes a chapter in New York's ongoing tale of endurance and elegance.

4. Bow Bridge Ballet: Poise, Posture, and Plies in the Park

In "Bow Bridge Ballet: Poise, Posture, and Plies in the Park," this chapter brings the elegance of ballet to the heart of Central Park, where dancers become part of Manhattan's iconic landscape. At the Bow Bridge, each pirouette and plie is a fusion of passion, precision, and poetry, creating a graceful harmony with the city's rhythm. Here, ballet is more than movement; it's a soulful expression, a way to connect with the romance and allure of the city. With every step, dancers craft their own story in The Manhattan Diaries, turning the park into a stage and Manhattan's skyline into their backdrop.

5. Sheep Meadow Yoga: Stretching Amidst the Skyscrapers' Silhouette

In "Sheep Meadow Yoga: Stretching Amidst the Skyscrapers' Silhouette," this chapter invites readers to experience yoga as a grounding force within Manhattan's dynamic energy. Set against the iconic skyline in Central Park's Sheep Meadow, each pose transforms into a serene moment of connection between the self and the city. Beyond stretching muscles, this practice stretches boundaries, harmonizing with the city's hum while embracing the openness of the meadow. Here, yoga becomes a meditative dance with the urban landscape, where every breath resonates with Manhattan's timeless spirit and every asana is an anthem within The Manhattan Diaries.

6. Belvedere Castle Climbs: Staircase Workouts for Royalty in Training

In "Belvedere Castle Climbs: Staircase Workouts for Royalty in Training," this chapter of The Manhattan Diaries transforms the ascent of Belvedere Castle into a regal workout experience, fusing fitness with the flair of royalty. Each step is more than a physical challenge; it's a tribute to Manhattan's grandeur, blending the city's historical weight with the elegance of a modern-day monarch. From slow, dignified climbs to swift, rhythmic strides, readers will discover how to elevate not only their fitness but also their spirit, mirroring the city's own lofty ambitions. Embrace the Manhattan rise, for in this city, every climb is a testament to strength, grace, and the pursuit of greatness.

7. Strawberry Fields Forever Fit: Toning to the Tunes of Legends

In "Strawberry Fields Forever Fit: Toning to the Tunes of Legends," this chapter of The Manhattan Diaries invites readers to experience the magic of toning their bodies to Manhattan's iconic music scene, where each movement is set to the city's legendary melodies. With Central Park West as the stage, fitness becomes a fusion of rhythm and history, harmonizing with Manhattan's musical legacy from timeless ballads to pop anthems. It's not only about sculpting muscles but connecting with the heartbeat of the city through dance, capturing the spirit of icons and embodying the energy of every beat. Lace up, find your rhythm, and step into the city's melodic embrace.

8. Conservatory Water Cardio: Rowing Your Way to Radiance

In "Conservatory Water Cardio: Rowing Your Way to Radiance," this chapter of The Manhattan Diaries delves into the art of rowing on Central Park's serene Conservatory Water, where each stroke tells a story of elegance and ambition. Here, rowing becomes a graceful "Manhattan Water Waltz" against the city's bustling backdrop, blending strength and style in perfect harmony. It's more than just a workout; it's about connecting with the rhythm of Manhattan itself, balancing the tranquility of Central Park's waters with the city's vibrant energy. With each pull of the oars, readers are invited to transform fitness into a poetic, aquatic ballet, embodying the grace and allure of the city.

9. Central Park West Heights: Lifting with the View of Penthouses

In "Central Park West Heights: Lifting with the View of Penthouses," this chapter of The Manhattan Diaries explores the art of strength training against the iconic backdrop of Central Park West's skyline. Here, each lift and squat is more than a workout—it's an experience that embodies Manhattan's energy, ambition, and elegance. Amidst towering penthouses and lush park views, the "Manhattan Weighted Waltz" transforms every rep into a powerful statement of purpose, merging the thrill of fitness with the city's grandeur. Readers are invited to embrace this elite workout, where every move brings them closer to sculpting not just their bodies but their own New York story.

10. The Ramble Routines: Fitness Trails Amidst Nature's Finest

"The Ramble Routines: Fitness Trails Amidst Nature's Finest" invites readers to discover the art of blending fitness with the serene beauty of Central Park's woodland haven, The Ramble. In this chapter of The Manhattan Diaries, every jog and sprint becomes a graceful journey, echoing Manhattan's dynamic pulse while syncing with the tranquility of nature. More than just a workout, it's a rhythmic experience that merges city sophistication with the wonder of untamed landscapes, reminding us that even in Manhattan's bustling heart, there's a sanctuary waiting to be explored. Each step, each breath, becomes part of the city's hidden symphony, transforming every trail into a path of purpose and reflection amidst nature's embrace.

Where Do We Go From Here?

In the heart of Manhattan's ceaseless energy, amidst the ever-evolving tales of ambition and allure, we find ourselves at a crossroads. "Where do we go from here?" This question, like the city itself, carries an air of anticipation and endless possibilities. As we've uncovered the secrets of "Central Park's Fitness Hacks" and reveled in the luxuries of Manhattan living, it's only natural to contemplate our next steps.

Manhattan, much like life itself, is a series of chapters waiting to be written. Each street, each skyline, each encounter has a story to tell, and we are the authors of our own Manhattan Diaries. From the tranquil moments in the park to the vibrant energy of the city's streets, we've discovered that every experience adds a unique hue to the canvas of our lives.

Manhattan, much like life itself, is a series of chapters waiting to be written. Each street, each skyline, each encounter has a story to tell, and we are the authors of our own Manhattan Diaries. From the tranquil moments in the park to the vibrant energy of the city's streets, we've discovered that every experience adds a unique hue to the canvas of our lives.

In "Rise and Shine, Manhattan-Style," the eighth book of The Manhattan Diaries, we'll delve into the day-to-day luxuries that make this city so extraordinary.

From savoring a perfectly brewed coffee while gazing at the city's iconic landmarks to the thrill of a spontaneous rooftop soirée, Manhattan offers a tapestry of experiences waiting to be embraced.

So, as we stand at this juncture, let us remember that the journey through Manhattan's mysteries is far from over. With each new day, we have the opportunity to explore, reinvent, and uncover facets of ourselves we never knew existed. Where do we go from here? The answer lies within the city's heartbeat, in its whispers of inspiration, and in the endless discoveries waiting to be made.

Let us embrace the next chapter with the same fervor that defines this city—because in Manhattan, the adventure never ends, and the possibilities are boundless.

Completed Tasks: Recap Checklist Activities

Inspirational Quote

IT DOES NOT MATTER HOW SLOWLY YOU GO AS LONG AS YOU DO NOT STOP. — Confucius

Action Items: Intentions and Thoughts

Journal Pages: Pen Your Tales

Journal Pages: Pen Your Tales

Journal Pages: Pen Your Tales

Journal Pages: Pen Your Tales

Journal Pages: Pen Your Tales

Journal Pages: Pen Your Tales

Journal Pages: Pen Your Tales

Journal Pages: Pen Your Tales

Journal Pages: Pen Your Tales

www.ingramcontent.com/pod-product-compliance
Lightning Source LLC
Chambersburg PA
CBHW032054020426
42335CB00011B/327